Stress

Key Issues in Mental Health

Vol. 174

Series Editors

A. Riecher-Rössler Basel

M. Steiner Hamilton

Stress
The Brain-Body Connection

Volume Editors

Dirk H. Hellhammer Trier
Juliane Hellhammer Trier

3 figures, 2008

KARGER

Basel · Freiburg · Paris · London · New York ·
Bangalore · Bangkok · Singapore · Tokyo · Sydney

Key Issues in Mental Health
Formerly published as 'Bibliotheca Psychiatrica' (founded 1917)

Dirk H. Hellhammer
Professor of Psychobiology
Trier University
Johanniterufer 15
DE–54290 Trier

Juliane Hellhammer
CEO, Daacro GmbH & Co. KG
Contract Research Organization
Novalisstrasse 12a
DE–54295 Trier

Disclosure Statement

We hereby state that Neuropattern is a registered trademark and that we are interested in making this diagnostic system commercially available for routine use in clinical practice.

Library of Congress Cataloging-in-Publication Data

Stress : the brain-body connection / volume editors, Dirk H. Hellhammer, Juliane Hellhammer.
p. ; cm. -- (Key issues in mental health, ISSN 1662-4874 ; v. 174)
Includes bibliographical references and index.
ISBN 978-3-8055-8295-7 (hard cover : alk. paper)
1. Stress (Psychology) 2. Mind and body. 3. Neuropsychology. I. Hellhammer, Dirk H. II. Hellhammer, Juliane. III. Series.
[DNLM: 1. Stress, Psychological–physiopathology. 2. Neurobehavioral Manifestations. 3. Psychophysiology–methods. 4. Sympathetic Nervous System–physiopathology. W172 S91582 2008 / WM 172 M663 2008]
RC455.4.S87S75 2008
616.9'8--dc22

2007051232

Bibliographic Indices. This publication is listed in bibliographic services, including Current Contents® and Index Medicus.

www.karger.com
Printed in Switzerland on acid-free and non-aging paper (ISO 9706) by Reinhardt Druck, Basel
ISSN 1662–4874
ISBN 978–3–8055–8295–7

Contents

Foreword

Stress refers to the process of adaptation of an individual once he/she is exposed to external or internal challenges. The organism possesses numerous systems to coordinate such adaptive responses, both at the systemic and the cellular level. In this book, we address stress-related bodily disorders, and, consequently, the mechanisms that participate in the crosstalk between the brain and the body; mainly the endocrine, the immune, and the autonomic nervous systems. Maladaptation may result in stress-related disorders, which eventually affect all organ systems and can involve central and peripheral mechanisms since this crosstalk is truly bi-directional.

Maladaptation to stress alters both brain function and peripheral physiology, and can promote a broad array of psychological (e.g. depression, burnout, anxiety and pain disorders) and somatic disturbances (e.g. cardiovascular, metabolic, reproductive, immunological, gastrointestinal, sensorimotor disorders). The risk of developing stress-related disorders or diseases is determined by a tremendous complexity of genetic and developmental factors, which varies strongly among individuals and sometimes even share similar symptoms. In addition, there is a lack of covariance between the psychological and the bodily stress responses. Thus, subjective reports from patients provide only poor information and may result in inappropriate diagnostic and therapeutic interventions.

Thus, the continuous increase of stress-related disorders in civilized countries and the rapid growth of knowledge on the psychobiological mechanisms behind them are challenging clinicians and researchers across different disciplines. This book first illustrates some aspects of the particular situation patients face once seeking help for stress-related disorders. We then introduce a new diagnostic strategy, which may help account for some of these challenges. This new method of assessing 'neuropatterns' has been created by Dirk Hellhammer and was developed at the University of Trier, Germany, by his research group. These neuropatterns specifically characterize and discriminate between the activities of interfaces, which participate in the adaptation of the endocrine and autonomic nervous system to stress. This diagnostic approach attempts to measure the activity of interfaces, which take part in the crosstalk between the brain and peripheral organs during adaptation to stress. The activity of these interfaces is assessed by concomitant biological, psychological, and symptomatic changes.

We here provide the first introduction to this method. All chapters are authored by members of the Trier research group, and they provide an update on how stress affects the brain-body connection. The clinical usefulness of this approach is exemplified with case studies. In order not to interfere with the readability of the text and to enable the reader to obtain introductory information on the subject, the authors have preferably cited only overviews and reviews from the relevant literature. Since the brain is part of the body, we are aware that the title of this book is a compromise to language use. 'Stress. The Brain-Body Connection' may best reflect what we are writing about.

Dirk H. Hellhammer, Juliane Hellhammer
Trier, Germany

Hellhammer DH, Hellhammer J (eds): Stress. The Brain-Body Connection.
Key Issues in Mental Health. Basel, Karger, 2008, vol 174, pp 1–10

1. Neurobehavioral Medicine and Stress-Related Disorders

Dirk H. Hellhammer · Juliane Hellhammer

Industrialized countries are being faced with an increasing burden of stress-related disorders. Lademann et al. [1] recently provided a meta-analysis of reports from German insurance companies, demonstrating a rapid increase in stress-related disorders in the last decade, as operationalized by missing work days. In addition, Andlin-Sobocki et al. [2] documented the tremendous financial burden arising as a consequence of stress-related disorders. Such data meet reports from the American Institute of Stress (AIS) estimating that workplace stress results in accidents, absenteeism, employee turnover, diminished productivity, direct medical, legal, and insurance costs, workers' compensation awards, etc., which sum up in the United States to more than USD 300 billion each year.

Following the same lines, the World Health Organization [3] documented an increasing prevalence of psychiatric disorders in Europe. According to that report, 33.4 million Europeans currently suffer a major depression in any given year, and mental health problems account for up to 30% of consultations with general practitioners in Europe. In one northern European member state, stress-related conditions account for more than half of all disabilities, while in one decade life expectancy has decreased by 10 years in some Member States, mainly due to stress and conditions related to mental ill health.

These and other reports clearly call for adequate strategies for the prevention and intervention of stress-related disorders. However, there is a big gap between basic research and clinical application. Over the last decades, countless research papers have been published on stress-related psychological, biological, and symptomatological relationships, but all this knowledge has only had a minor impact for the patient. Obviously, the time is ripe to bridge this gap and, currently, several interesting strategies and approaches exist, which are relevant for stress medicine.

1.1. Strategies to Bridge the Gap between Bench and Bedside

Both the above-mentioned situation and the rapid increase of knowledge from the biosciences call for new strategies to improve medical care. We will briefly address some of the most relevant and promising recent approaches.

1.1.1. Translational Research

The National Institutes of Health (NIH) recently released a roadmap program. The respective website [4] summarizes the intentions of this program: 'To improve human health, scientific discoveries must be translated into practical applications. Such discoveries typically begin at "the bench" with basic research – in which scientists study disease at a molecular or cellular level – then progress to the clinical level, or the patient's "bedside". Scientists are increasingly aware that this bench-to-bedside approach to translational research is really a two-way street. Basic scientists provide clinicians with new tools for use in patients and for assessment of their impact, and clinical researchers make novel observations about the nature and progression of disease that often stimulate basic investigations. Translational research has proven to be a powerful process that drives the clinical research engine. However, a stronger research infrastructure could strengthen and accelerate this critical part of the clinical research enterprise. The NIH roadmap attempts to catalyze translational research in various ways. (...) The challenge is how do we deal with the massive amount of information that comes from gene sequencing, gene expression, proteomic data, and metabolomics on the one hand, and connect that to data from a particular patient?'

Thus, the barriers of translational research are evident – not only by the increasing complexity of information but also from practical issues. Conducting clinical trials is another challenge in itself, and both limit professional interest in the field and hamper the clinical research enterprise.

With respect to stress-related disorders, another specific trans-NIH initiative has recently been announced by the NIH, which has been named 'MUSIC' (the Medically Unexplained Syndrome Institutional Collaborative): 'Medically unexplained syndromes (MUS) present the most common problems in medicine. Most medical specialties treat (at least one) MUS; e.g. urologists treat interstitial cystitis, gastroenterologists treat irritable bowel syndrome, gynecologists treat chronic pelvic pain, rheumatologists treat chronic fatigue syndrome and fibromyalgia, psychiatrists treat panic disorder, etc. Specialists generally treat these patients in relative isolation, without consideration of the potentially confounding influence(s) of the frequently overlapping comorbid disorders their patients suffer.' The NIH expects that this initiative has the potential 'to dramatically affect how biomedical and behavioral research is conducted over the next decade for the benefit of public health' [5].

1.1.2. Early Adversity

The impact of pre- and postnatal adversity on mood and anxiety disorders has recently been reviewed comprehensively in this series [6]. With respect to stress-related disorders, this field has been stimulated tremendously by the pathfinding observations of Seymour Levine and David Barker, and, with respect to neurobiological mechanisms, by Michael Meaney, Stephen Matthews, Charles Nemeroff, Paul Plotsky, Jonathan Seckl and Steven Suomi. These and many other researchers provided evidence that the brain and other organs respond very sensitively to the maternal and postnatal environment across different stages of development. Such effects permanently alter the ability of individuals to adapt to stress in later life, and lead them to eventually develop stress-related disorders such as abdominal obesity, type 2 diabetes, cardiovascular disease, irritable bowel syndrome, etc. (for reviews, see [7–11]). Pre- and postnatal programming seems to be most relevant for stress vulnerability in later life. The chapters in this volume will demonstrate this in more detail.

1.1.3. Genetics and Epigenetics

The Human Genome Project has strongly stimulated research on stress-related disorders. Attempts have been undertaken to identify specific genes and their associated gene activities, e.g. in patients who have chronic fatigue syndrome (CFS) [12], while Heim et al. [13] showed evidence of increased levels of multiple types of childhood trauma in a population-based sample of clinically confirmed CFS cases. It is not unlikely that gene expression is differentially affected by trauma in CFS patients, and that disease onset occurs once both risk factors are added. Gene × environment interactions have been illustrated nicely for human depression [14], posttraumatic stress disorder [15], anxiety disorders [16], as well as for the epigenetic mechanisms behind them [17]. However, this kind of research is rather recent and, for stress-related bodily disorders, studies on gene × environment interactions have only just begun.

1.1.4. Behavioral Neurobiology

Research in both animals and people has focused on brain mechanisms involved in stress, depression, anxiety and concomitant bodily responses. New methods such as knock-out mice and transgenic mice models and neuroimaging have been introduced, all resulting in a rapid increase of knowledge on how the brain determines behavior and how behavior affects the brain. Research studies that focus on the role of prefrontal cortex in the regulation of emotions are a good example for this. Imaging studies in both monkeys and humans resulted in models which provide a very conclusive view of the brain areas involved [18, 19]. On the basis of this knowledge it now seems possible to manipulate these brain areas using new technologies [20], such as photostimulation.

1.1.5. Individualized Interventions

Research studies in biological psychiatry and psychology are usually deductive and empirical, while it is difficult to get funding and acceptance for publication of case studies. However, in a given patient with stress-related disorders, etiological and pathogenic factors are always complex and thus rather unique. This calls for individualized diagnostic and therapeutic interventions.

To promote this strategy, the Association for Patient-Oriented Research (APOR) has been founded, which considers patient-oriented research to be a core discipline of medicine. APOR attempts to strengthen the education of clinical investigators and advocates support for patient-oriented clinical research.

In addition, the Food and Drug Administration in the USA recently issued two initiatives, which could prove seminal in establishing personalized medicine as a key part of drug development and healthcare. Personalized medicine can be defined as being the ability to individualize therapy by predicting which individuals have a greater chance of benefit or risk, helping to maximize the drug safety and effectiveness. This relies upon the ability to identify key biomarkers associated with a particular disease or disease subgroup and the availability of treatment for the particular disease. In addition, the physician should be helped to identify the markers in a particular subject to effectively match the treatment. Personalized medicine is strongly supported by another NIH roadmap program (www.nihroadmap.nih.gov/molecularlibraries).

Psychotherapists probably know best about the necessity of individualized treatments for stress-related disorders. However, their therapeutic approaches are usually not based on psychobiological research, and pharmacological treatments are poorly personalized. Grawe [21] put forward a claim for what he called 'neuropsychotherapy' to improve psychotherapy by incorporating knowledge from the neurosciences. In the past decade, quite a few research studies have been undertaken to apply imaging techniques to monitor the effects of psychotherapy [22, 23], and to improve the integration of psychotherapeutic and pharmacotherapeutic treatments for most psychiatric and neurological disorders. Some of this research as well as a couple of studies on stress-related disorders will be addressed in the chapters of this volume.

Other strategies try to incorporate knowledge on the mechanisms which could finally not only allow to monitoring a psychobiological process but also to control it. Such an approach has been taken up by the International Society of Psychoneuroendocrinology (ISPNE). The new 'Brain-Body-Initiative' (BBI) of ISPNE, drafted by Michael Meaney, promotes a transdisciplinary model of research that respects multiple levels of analysis and explanation, literally from the sociological to the genetic, and bridges the conceptual divide that separates the disciplines. Knowledge transfer will be achieved through the development of e-based educational programs and publications. A virtual network of leading scientists worldwide and members of partner organizations and expert working groups attempting to identify innovative research programs, as well as scientists at the interface of the physical, biological, and social sciences will define the relation between gene × environment interactions – neurophenotypes – illness and recovery from illness.

In summary, all these strategies target a patient-oriented transfer of neurobiological knowledge to improve diagnostic and therapeutic interventions. Most of this research is done in the area of biological psychiatry and neuropsychopharmacology. Only recently has this type of strategic approach been extended to behavioral medicine by initiatives such as MUSIC and BBI. Thus, psychosomatic medicine or behavioral medicine may merge and constitute a new area, which could be called neurobehavioral medicine.

1.2. Neurobehavioral Medicine

Different disciplines such as psychosomatic medicine, behavioral medicine, and health psychology attempt to understand the behavioral and biomedical correlates of such disorders. Behavioral medicine focuses primarily on the prevention, diagnosis, treatment, and rehabilitation of these and other disturbances [24, 25], while health psychology is additionally directed towards the promotion of health behavior [26]. Psychosomatic medicine had more favors in the understanding of specific psychobiological mechanisms which may be causally associated with such disorders [27].

Over the past decades, a wide knowledge has been accumulated from all these different disciplines. Clinically oriented research resulted in an improvement of the promotion, prevention, diagnosis, therapy, and rehabilitation of specific disorders. However, there is a tremendous amount of knowledge about neurobiological mechanisms participating in and possibly causing bodily disturbances that has rarely been incorporated in the clinical routine. Only recently have clinical translational programs been developed, targeting neurobehavioral medicine as an extended integrative discipline with the goal of developing a systematic approach to understanding the complex interactions between psychological, neuronal, endocrinological and immunological factors which could possibly promote or cause psychosomatic disorders. Historically, a very first approach to integrate neurobiological and psychological processes with symptom formation was already attempted by Freud in 1895 [28]. In a later analysis of his 'Project for a Scientific Psychology' Pribram and Gill [29, p.10] showed 'that Freud initially formulated the mechanisms of mental function on the basis of his biological and neurological knowledge.' In the second half of the last century, Weiner [30] pioneered the field by his landmarking book *Psychobiology and Human Disease*. Today, we have learned to accept that neuronal, endocrine, and immune processes associated with stress-related disorders are tremendously complex. Fortunately, considerable research from neurobiology and medicine is available to conceptualize at least some of these mechanisms. Such concepts are important to create interdisciplinary dialogues and data exchange, thus establishing the basis needed for neurobehavioral medicine.

The search for mechanisms per se is conceptual, since it often implies the transfer of knowledge from animal or human experiments to the clinical situation. The degree of conceptualization, however, may vary considerably. If we are seriously interested in investigating the psychobiological mechanisms that promote or cause bodily disorders, we need to refer to knowledge from animals and humans from very different disciplines such as the social and behavioral sciences, neurobiology, biochemistry, physiology, and clinical medicine. Most of these subjects comprise numerous highly specialized subfields (i.e. psychotherapy, molecular neurobiology, gynecology, dermatology, neuroendocrinology, immunology, gastroenterology, oncology, etc.). This specialization as well as divergent research interests make it very difficult to establish an interdisciplinary communication among these very different disciplines.

It is a major task of neurobehavioral medicine to investigate the behavioral and biological mechanisms relevant for the etiology and pathogenesis of bodily disorders. The necessity of interdisciplinary research creates the need of models, which allow conceptualizing the specific neuroendocrine mechanisms participating in stress-related disorders. Such theoretical models may serve as valuable tools not only to integrate the heuristic knowledge from divergent research areas, but also to functionally link these data. Obviously, these models will be highly speculative and risky, and they may, at least in part, be entirely wrong. However, the hypotheses derived from these models will be testable. The delivery of testable hypotheses is another important benefit of such models.

Conceptual approaches are not limited to enabling researchers to develop a deeper understanding of specific psychobiological mechanisms in stress-related disorders. They may also create new general insights into behaviorally induced brain processes that modulate the communication between the nervous, endocrine, and immune systems. It is possible that specific neuroendophenotypes will be discovered that are relevant for several somatic disturbances (to see this from an evolutionary perspective, see Panksepp [31]). This may be an important step, since it will extend our conceptual approaches from clinical symptomatology to clinical psychobiology.

We can speculate that the application of neurobehavioral medicine will yield new types of information. For example, descriptions of psychobiological complexities in different disorders may first lead to the finding that some general mechanisms exist, which are used by the brain to adapt peripheral physiological function to the status of stress. Secondly, we have to expect that observable behavioral and physiological symptoms occur as a consequence of specific brain activities. If so, an adequate interpretation of symptoms may demand psychobiological rather than psychological explanations. Furthermore, we may learn more about brain processes such as the generation of rhythms and self-regulatory mechanisms on the molecular, cellular and organ levels relevant for our understanding of principles by which the brain processes these stressful events. Thus, it will be a specific task of neurobehavioral medicine to document and conceptualize brain processes and the resulting behavioral and

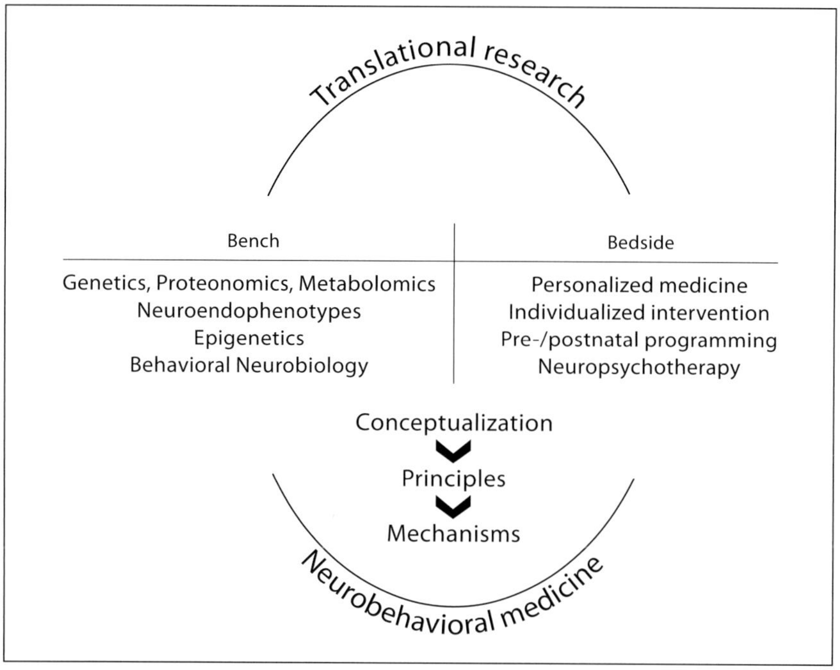

Fig. 1.1. Elements of neurobehavioral medicine.

bodily events to obtain adequate descriptions of the psychobiological mechanisms involved in stress-related disorders.

Furthermore, it may be helpful to identify the general principles of the crosstalk between the brain and the body. These principles may provide guidance and increase translational efficacy. Such principles should refer to adaptation to stress (fig. 1.1.). In chapter 3, we describe those principles which characterize adaptation, namely glandotropy, ergothropy, and trophotropy.

In summary, neurobehavioral medicine may attempt to extend behavioral medicine by understanding the language of the brain in the processing of psychological and behavioral events. We feel that there is a treasury of knowledge to be gained from the neurosciences, which can already be of benefit for behavioral medicine. Brain systems have their own mode of determining psychological and biological events as well as communication with other organs. We need to understand the language of these systems to perceive how the organism adapts to stress, and how maladaptation causes somatic disorders. For a meaningful interdisciplinary exchange of data, it is necessary to take the risk of integrating the present knowledge within the available models. Testable hypotheses derived from such models may facilitate interdisciplinary exchange and research. Thus, conceptual psychobiology is an essential tool for neurobehavioral medicine.

1.3. Conclusions

The behavioral and health scientists may not yet feel an urgent need for neurobehavioral medicine, and some may doubt that the time has already come (or may ever come) for a clinically efficient integration of both the behavioral sciences and the neurosciences. This debate is also relevant for biological psychiatry. For example, our knowledge on brain mechanisms participating in anxiety or depression is very comprehensive, and many studies detected meaningful relationships between clinical symptoms and biological alterations [32]. On the other hand, there is a tremendous amount of research from the clinical sciences, and very-well-documented data on the importance of social and psychological variables in the etiology and pathogenesis of depression [33–35]. Thus, both research areas have contributed independently and profoundly to our understanding of these disorders. But it has become obvious that neither the biological nor the clinical sciences alone will be able to solve the enigma of these disorders. Interdisciplinary research from biological psychiatry has proven to considerably improve our knowledge on such disorders, and it seems that mind-body-medicine can also profit from interdisciplinary research [27]. Such an interdisciplinary approach can become very stimulating and may provide valuable guidance for new research projects. In this sense, neurobehavioral models serve as research tools and do not claim to provide final answers to any given question. Thus, we believe that the time is ripe and that there is no good alternative to this type of developmental approach.

The various participating disciplines can contribute very specific pieces obtained by very specific methodology but, again, this may not be sufficient to place all the pieces of the jigsaw puzzle together. In addition, neurobehavioral medicine has to develop its own repertoire of research methods. With respect to diagnostics, we already mentioned that knowledge about specific brain functions can help discriminate different pathological mechanisms in different subgroups of patients. Therapeutic strategies may also benefit from neurobehavioral medicine. Based on our concepts of the psychobiology of the respective disorders, we may be able to find the most efficient approach to combine social, psychological, and medical interventions for the treatment of subgroups.

1.4. Summary

Our knowledge on the brain processes involved in stress and stress pathology has rapidly increased during the past decades. Today, the time is ripe for a neurobehavioral medicine based on genetics, proteonomics, metabolomics, epigenetic, and behavioral neurobiology. To bridge the gap between bench and bedside, one has to conceptualize and integrate this knowledge at different levels, ranging from neurophenotypes to principles of physiological processes participating in the adaptation to stress.

Obviously, strong interest in individualized interventions and pre- to postnatal programming of stress vulnerability currently emerges, which may constitute a major translational research goal in the near future.

References

1 Lademann J, Mertesacker H, Gebhardt B: Psychische Erkrankungen im Fokus der Gesundheitsreporte der Krankenkassen. Psychotherapeutenjournal 2006;5:123–129.

2 Andlin-Sobocki P, Jonsson B, Wittchen HU, Olesen J: Cost of disorders of the brain in Europe. Eur J Neurol 2005;12(suppl 1):1–27.

3 WHO: Mental Health in the WHO European Region; in: Fact sheet EURO. Geneva, World Health Organization, 2003.

4 Translational Research: National Institute of Health (NIH), 2007. (Accessed 07/15/07, at http://nihroadmap.nih.gov/clinicalresearch/overview-translational.asp.)

5 NIH Roadmap for Medical Research: National Institutes of Health, 2006. (Accessed 11/05/2006, 2006, at http://nihroadmap.nih.gov/.)

6 Riecher-Rössler A, Steiner M: Perinatal Stress, Mood and Anxiety Disorders: From Bench to Bedside. Basel, Karger, 2005.

7 Barker DJ: The developmental origins of chronic adult disease. Acta Paediatr Suppl 2004;93:26–33.

8 Francis DD, Caldji C, Champagne F, Plotsky PM, Meaney MJ: The role of corticotropin-releasing factor-norepinephrine systems in mediating the effects of early experience on the development of behavioral and endocrine responses to stress. Biol Psychiatry 1999;46:1153–1166.

9 Heim C, Plotsky PM, Nemeroff CB: Importance of studying the contributions of early adverse experience to neurobiological findings in depression. Neuropsychopharmacology 2004;29:641–648.

10 Phillips DI, Jones A: Fetal programming of autonomic and HPA function: do people who were small babies have enhanced stress responses? J Physiol 2006;572:45–50.

11 Seckl JR, Meaney MJ: Glucocorticoid programming. Ann NY Acad Sci 2004;1032:63–84.

12 Kerr JR, Christian P, Hodgetts A, Langford PR, Devanur LD, Petty R, Burke B, Sinclair LI, Richards SC, Montgomery J, McDermott CR, Harrison TJ, Kellam P, Nutt DJ, Holgate ST, Group CCS: Current research priorities in chronic fatigue syndrome/myalgic encephalomyelitis: disease mechanisms, a diagnostic test and specific treatments. J Clin Pathol 2007;60:113–116.

13 Heim C, Wagner D, Maloney E, Papanicolaou DA, Solomon L, Jones JF, Unger ER, Reeves WC: Early adverse experience and risk for chronic fatigue syndrome: results from a population-based study. Arch Gen Psychiatry 2006;63:1258–1266.

14 Caspi A, Moffitt TE: Gene-environment interactions in psychiatry: joining forces with neuroscience. Nat Rev 2006;7:583–590.

15 Seckl JR, Meaney MJ: Glucocorticoid 'programming' and PTSD risk. Ann NY Acad Sci 2006;1071:351–378.

16 Gross C, Hen R: Genetic and environmental factors interact to influence anxiety. Neurotox Res 2004;6:493–501.

17 Meaney MJ, Szyf M: Environmental programming of stress responses through DNA methylation: life at the interface between a dynamic environment and a fixed genome. Dialog Clin Neurosci 2005;7:103–123.

18 Davidson RJ: Anxiety and affective style: role of prefrontal cortex and amygdala. Biol Psychiatry 2002;51:68–80.

19 Mayberg H: Depression. II. Localization of pathophysiology. Am J Psychiatry 2002;159:1979.

20 Deisseroth K, Feng G, Majewska AK, Miesenbock G, Ting A, Schnitzer MJ: Next-generation optical technologies for illuminating genetically targeted brain circuits. J Neurosci 2006;26:10380–10386.

21 Grawe K: Neuropsychotherapy: How the Neurosciences Inform Effective Psychotherapy. Florence, Ky, Lawrence Erlbaum, 2006.

22 Linden D: How psychotherapy changes the brain: the contribution of functional neuroimaging. Mol Psychiatry 2006;11:528–538.

23 Etkin A, Pittenger C, Polan HJ, Kandel ER: Toward a neurobiology of psychotherapy: basic science and clinical applications. J Neuropsychiatry Clin Neurosci 2005;17:145–158.

24 Schwartz GE, Weiss SM: Yale Conference on Behavioral Medicine: a proposed definition and statement of goals. J Behav Med 1978;1:3–12.

25 Pomerleau O, Pertschuk M, Adkins D, Brady JP: A comparison of behavioral and traditional treatment for middle-income problem drinkers. J Behav Med 1978;1:187–200.

26 Matarazzo JD: Behavioral health and behavioral medicine: frontiers for a new health psychology. Am Psychol 1980;35:807–817.

27 Selhub EM: Stress and distress in clinical practice: a mind-body approach. Nutr Clin Care 2002;5:182–190.
28 Freud S: Project for a scientific psychology (1895); in: The Standard Edition of the Complete Psychological Works of Sigmund Freud. London, Hogarth Press, 1953, pp 283–397.
29 Pribram KH, Gill MM: Freud's Project Reassessed. New York, Basic Books, 1976.
30 Weiner H: Psychobiology and Human Disease. New York, Elsevier, 1977.
31 Panksepp J: Emotional endophenotypes in evolutionary psychiatry. Prog Neuro-Psychopharmacol Biol Psychiatry 2006;30:774–784.
32 McEwen BS: Physiology and neurobiology of stress and adaptation: central role of the brain. Physiol Rev 2007;87:873–904.
33 Hirschfeld RM, Montgomery SA, Keller MB, Kasper S, Schatzberg AF, Moller HJ, Healy D, Baldwin D, Humble M, Versiani M, Montenegro R, Bourgeois M: Social functioning in depression: a review. J Clin Psychiatry 2000;61:268–275.
34 Billings AG, Moos RH: Coping, stress, and social resources among adults with unipolar depression. J Pers Soc Psychol 1984;46:877–891.
35 Mirowsky J, Ross CE: Social Causes of Psychological Distress, ed 2. Hawthorne, Gruyter, 2003.

Hellhammer DH, Hellhammer J (eds): Stress. The Brain-Body Connection.
Key Issues in Mental Health. Basel, Karger, 2008, vol 174, pp 11–20

2. Neuropattern – A Step towards Neurobehavioral Medicine

Dirk H. Hellhammer · Juliane Hellhammer

In chapter 1, we argued that the time is ripe for what one may call 'neurobehavioral medicine'. However, 'bench-to-bed' strategies have rarely been applied to stress-related disorders. Thus, we here address the criteria that need to be fulfilled by a systematic clinical translational approach in neurobehavioral medicine. We will then introduce 'Neuropattern', a new and recently developed diagnostic tool that meets these criteria.

2.1. Criteria for Clinical Translational Diagnostics

We think that a useful diagnostic system has to account for the following criteria:

- Complexity and heterogeneity of etiopathogenetic mechanisms in stress-related disorders.
- Missing covariance of psychological and biological measures of the stress response.
- Being translational by applying state-of-the-art psychobiological knowledge to clinical treatment.
- Being easily accessible to practitioners in primary care, specialists, and across different disciplines in hospitals.
- Allowing a permanent exchange and update of data generated from basic research and bedside results.
- Improving therapeutic success and cost-effectiveness.

These issues will be addressed below and we will try to identify a strategy which may help develop such a diagnostic tool.

2.1.1. Complexity and Heterogeneity

Several bodily disturbances are considered to be psychosomatic since their onset and reoccurrence seems to be influenced by psychological, social, or behavioral events. For hypertension, for example, psychological factors such as anger and aggression, social status, or type A behavior have been discussed as relevant determinants of high blood pressure [1, 2]. However, many other factors, such as prenatal programming, cholesterol, family history, sex, race, gene polymorphisms, high-sodium diet, age, obesity, excessive smoking and alcohol consumption have also been considered important risk factors [3–6].

If we think about mechanisms, several questions become relevant. The first question concerns the specificity of psychological or behavioral events that can by themselves evoke the symptomatology. If this is not the case, we have to ask if other risk factors play a role, and if a complexity of risk factors is characteristic for a subgroup of patients, or if such complexities are unspecific. If a specific pattern exists, the question again is if the respective disorder is a casual or an indispensable consequence of such an interaction of risk factors. In other words, some subjects may be able to mobilize protective factors, counteracting these risk factors, thus staying healthy. Furthermore, it is necessary to find out if psychological, social, or behavioral risk factors are mandatory within such a cluster, or if they simply coexist without having any pathological relevance [7].

Given the fact that patterns of events causing disease do not occur randomly, it will be helpful to discriminate between subgroups of patients. These subgroups can be characterized by a specific functional interaction of risk factors. Such patterns may either comprehend several biological risk factors or behavioral risk factors interacting with biological factors. Furthermore, it is not unlikely that even in patients with rather homologous symptoms, heterogeneous subgroups can be defined. Some of them may solely include patterns of biological but others additional behavioral risk factors, and this knowledge is highly relevant for the correct diagnostic and differential diagnostic treatments.

We thus have to expect that each patient has a highly individual constellation of biological and psychological determinants of his/her disease. These determinants interact, which results in secondary or tertiary effects, and they may become clinically relevant depending on the interplay between genes and the environment. Facing such a tremendous complexity and heterogeneity of mechanisms in stress-related disorders, we have to ask if and how it will be possible to account for them in clinical routine. It will simply be impossible for a practitioner to overlook the variety of all these factors, and it will be unaffordable to apply the necessary measures, such as combinations of gene chips, imaging, etc. Even if all this would be possible, our present knowledge is not yet sufficient to fully uncover and intervene with the etiopathogenetic mechanisms in a given patient. Finally, we are learning day by day about new mechanisms likely to be relevant for stress-related disorders. Does this mean that we are overstressed and have to give up looking for individualized or personalized treatments?

2.1.2. Missing Covariance

One of the most neglected realities in stress medicine is the profound dissociation between the psychological and the bodily stress response. In other words: while some patients perceive high psychological stress without emitting a peripheral physiological stress response, others show strong physiological arousal without perceiving stress. What does it mean in practice? If a patient sees a doctor, the diagnostic treatment and the therapeutic decision will largely depend on the complaints the patient reports. Patients with stress-related disorders, however, may report wrongly to the physician, and thus receive an inappropriate treatment. The reason for this is that patients are likely to be unable to correctly perceive – and thus report – a relationship between their psychological and physiological stress responses. One patient, for example, feels severely stressed and reports his somatic symptoms as a consequence of stress, although this may clearly be wrong. The other patient may show pronounced somatic symptoms, but does not subjectively perceive and report stress. In both cases, patient reports are misleading, and the diagnostic and therapeutic treatment will most likely be inadequate.

Thus, we have to expect that both patients and therapists conceptualize stress-related disorders wrongly. Since the brain controls the outflow to the endocrine and autonomic nervous system, it is routinely assumed that physiological stress responses are largely modulated by psychological factors involved in the perception and appraisal of stressors [8]. However, while this has been demonstrated on the psychological and behavioral levels, such a covariance is rarely observed for peripheral physiological responses.

This lack of covariance has been known for many decades: Forty years ago, Lacey [9] wrote: 'There are many experimental results that sharply contradict activation theory. They cannot be discussed as due to sampling errors, or to poor experimental control, or to unreliability of measurement. I think the experiments show that electroencephalographic, autonomic, motor, and other behavioral systems are imperfectly coupled, complexly interacting systems. (...) I think the evidence also shows that one cannot easily use one form of arousal as a highly valid index of another.' While numerous research projects have addressed the 'covariance problem' in the past decades, it is not yet fully understood.

In an unpublished meta-analysis of data from our laboratory, which have been generated from hundreds of subjects exposed to the 'Trier Social Stress Test' (TSST), we could confirm a missing covariance among the psychological (state anxiety, mood, controllability, predictability, novelty, failure, etc.) and the biological (ACTH, plasma and salivary cortisol, glucocorticoid sensitivity, epinephrine, norepinephrine, blood pressure, heart rate, GH and prolactin, etc.) response measures. In his dissertation, Schlotz [10] recently illustrated this phenomenon for cortisol measures. Likewise, Fahrenberg [11] (translated by the authors) summarized that 'in contrast to the expected convergence of psychological (introspective, verbal) and physiological measures, empirical data generally yielded insignificant or weak correlations.

This divergence in the levels of analysis calls for a revision of theoretical concepts and the development and consequent application of multimodal diagnostics and evaluation.'

How can the lack of covariance be understood? How is it that several studies report covariance and show that psychological interventions (e.g. biofeedback, relaxation) dampen the physiological stress response and somatic symptoms? Probably, the brain processes a stressor on different levels of consciousness. Oversimplified, one may discriminate three response types, which all serve the organism to cope with a stressor:

(1) The immediate stress response: This response is characterized by an immediate mobilization of the autonomic nervous system and the hypothalamus-pituitary-adrenal axis (HPAA), and allows the organism to quickly emit a fight or flight response in the face of a threat. One may assume that this response is mainly controlled by subcortical mechanisms, e.g. from the diencephalon, the midbrain and the brainstem, and is thus largely unconscious and independent of the (subjective) perception of stress.

(2) The adaptive stress response: This response is characterized by adaptation to secondary signals from the body and the brain, which have been instantly activated by the stressor. It is directed towards perceived or anticipated threats of self-integrity, uncontrollability, uncertainty and novelty, and allows the individual to adequately adapt or habituate to these challenges. The adaptive stress response mainly involves allocortical brain structures such as the hippocampus and the amygdala, which, in part, also control those brain systems that modulate the immediate stress response. Physiological stress responsivity can be affected by adaptation and habituation. However, these processes may only partly be perceived consciously, and patient reports may predominantly refer to emotions, such as fear, anxiety, depression, and affective components of self-esteem.

(3) The evaluative stress response: This response is characterized by cognitive processes by which an individual responds (immediately and/or persistently) to an acute or chronic stressor. Cognitive processes refer to memories, associations, decision-making, etc., and mainly involve (neo-)cortical structures and pathways. The evaluative stress response may be uncoupled from the physiological stress response. Thus, a patient may perceive stress without emitting concomitant physiological and symptomatic responses. However, the adaptive stress response and, subsequently, the endocrine and autonomic outflow to the body may be affected indirectly.

This simplified discrimination of stress responses may illustrate that a missing covariance between perceived (conscious) stress and bodily stress responses is not always mandatory but rather likely. The exceptions are probably physiological responses of the brain, as verified by neuroimaging. For detailed descriptions of the functional neuroanatomy of stress, we refer to reviews by Herman et al. [12], Lopez et al. [13], Paczak and Palkovits [14], Charmandari et al. [15], Dallman et al. [16], and McEwen [17].

Missing covariance of the psychological and biological stress response is a characteristic and expected feature, and is probably also true for visceral perception [10]. The message from this research is that physicians cannot rely solely on patient reports if they want to diagnose stress-related disorders appropriately. This is a tremendous challenge for stress medicine.

2.1.3. Translational Concepts

In the past decade, numerous activities from research organizations and scientific societies as well as many publications have been released addressing the necessity of translational research. The different initiatives mentioned in chapter 1 and a recent publication from Porges [18] are good examples. In his editorial of the first issue of the *Journal of Translational Medicine* Marincola [19] states: 'The purpose of translational research is to test, in humans, novel therapeutic strategies developed through experimentation. Translational research should be regarded as a two-way road: bench-to-bedside and bedside-to-bench. However, bedside-to-bench efforts have regrettably been limited because the scientific aspects are poorly understood by full-time clinicians and the difficulty of dealing with humans poorly appreciated by basic scientists.'

For stress-related disorders, this situation is even worse for most practitioners, since stress medicine is not an area of general expertise. Today, translational approaches are mostly academic, and clinical application has not yet turned out to be satisfactory. It seems unrealistic to assume that practitioners could even acquire the necessary expertise, since such an education would be far too comprehensive to be included into curricula at universities or by continuous education. Thus, such a challenge calls for other unconventional strategies, separating expertise from clinical accessibility.

2.1.4. Accessibility to Clinical Routine

All of the previous challenges addressed here demand a strategy allowing the practitioner to access and handle expert knowledge. Not even psychiatrists or psychotherapists would be able to cope with the complexity, heterogeneity, and missing covariance of stress-related disorders once they attempt the translational approaches. On the other hand, experts in stress medicine would be unable to cover the clinical demands, as described in chapter 1.

In addition, stress may best be assessed under naturalistic conditions so that the measures have relatively high ecological validity [20]. A group of European scientists has recently created a network for ambulatory assessment (http://www.ambulatory-assessment.de), addressing the benefits of such an approach: 'Individual differences in behavior and physiology as well as behavior disorders and somatic symptoms are investigated in real-life situations where subjective state and relevant behavior can be studied much more effectively than in the artificial environment of laboratory research or with retrospective questionnaires.' Thus, stress-related measures may preferably be taken by noninvasive ambulatory methods, such as psychophysiological recordings and saliva sampling for hormone analyses.

These data, together with medical information provided by the physician, should then become available for expert analysis. To facilitate compliance of the physician, this implies a suited time management, which can be supported by adapting the available computer systems to allow quick transfer of medical data such as medical history. This may create a situation which would strongly facilitate a routine application in clinical practice.

2.1.5. Exchange and Update of Data

Exchanging data between bench and bedside will be necessary, since both basic research and clinical treatment can only benefit from learning from each other. Such a continuous feedback is mandatory to test the clinical efficacy of current concepts and to improve and scientifically update translational concepts and methods. Thus, it seems necessary to establish possibilities to collect and analyze the data and to elaborate on continuous updates.

2.1.6. Therapeutic Advantages and Cost-Effectiveness

If the criteria mentioned above are not fulfilled, two consequences seem to occur: First, the practitioners will be unable to reliably detect the impact of stress. Thus, they will often miss initiating an adequate therapeutic treatment. Indeed, it has been shown that patients with stress-related disorders often need years to get the necessary psychotherapeutic interventions [21, 22], and pharmacotherapeutic treatments frequently follow the trial and error paradigm [23, 24]. Second, even if the impact of stress becomes obvious, both pharmacotherapeutic and psychotherapeutic indications should be coordinated and adapted to the disease model. If there is no correct model, however, the therapeutic and cost-effectiveness will still be weak.

2.2. Neuropattern

In the past years, we have tried to develop a tool which meets the criteria mentioned above:

(1) To account for missing covariance, we decided to solely focus on the interfaces, which participate in the crosstalk between the brain and the body. These interfaces refer to different parts of the body which constitute the pituitary adrenal axis, and the autonomic nervous system as well as those brain nuclei which directly correspond with these systems under stress conditions. Since the activity of these interfaces implies covariance, we by-pass the issue of missing covariance.

(2) We then asked what we know from available research data about these interfaces. We conceptualized this knowledge for the status of hyper- and hypoactivity and reactivity for each interface. Using such a restrictive approach, we drastically reduced

the complexity issue, since we only worry about the activity or reactivity status of these interfaces, but not about the complex and heterogeneous determinants behind.

(3) To translate the knowledge to a practical but temporary diagnostic tool, we conceptualized three principles of brain-body communication under stress: the glandotropic, the ergotropic, and the trophotropic scenario (see chapters 3–7). The glandotropic scenario comprehends the activity and reactivity status of the paraventricular nucleus, the pituitary, and the adrenals, as well as the status of glucocorticoid receptor function. The ergotropic scenario includes the activity and reactivity status of the locus coeruleus and the sympathetic nervous system, while the trophotropic scenario mainly comprehends the raphe nuclei and the parasympathetic nervous system.

(4) To allow for application in clinical routine, we developed a kit containing questionnaires and devices for physiological measures:

(a) NPQ-A: Neuropattern questionnaire for amnestic data to be completed by the physician. The questionnaire records medical history, present treatments, medical data (blood pressure, heart rate, waist-to-hip ratio, etc.) and diagnoses.

(b) NPQ-B: Neuropattern questionnaire to be completed by the patient at home, including subjective reports on symptoms, disease development, symptom-free periods, treatments and treatment success, etc.

(c) NPQ-P: Neuropattern questionnaire to be completed by the patient at home, asking for all the specific psychological and further symptom variables, which have been assigned to the status of single interfaces.

(d) NP-PSQ: Neuropattern pre-, peri-, postnatal stress questionnaire, to be filled out by the patient at home, assisted by parents' information and birth records.

(e) Saliva collection: Saliva samples are collected at home or at the workplace on three consecutive workdays at awakening, and 30, 45 and 60 min later. On the evening of the second day, the patients take 0.25 mg dexamethasone to test for feedback sensitivity on the next day. During the first 2 days, additional samples are collected after lunch and at 8 p.m.

(f) Ambulatory autonomic measures: Estimates of sympathetic and parasympathetic activity are computed from heart rate variability measurements under controlled respiratory conditions by a portable device under resting conditions and a Schellong test. These measures are collected by the patients themselves at home or at the workplace.

(g) PHQ: Psychopathological conditions (e.g. anxiety and depression) are recorded by the PHQ (Patient Health Questionnaire) [25, 26].

(5) All data are posted to our laboratory. Here, the data of psychological, biological and symptom measures are analyzed and assigned to the respective neuropatterns. A neuropattern is an endophenotype characterizing the activity or reactivity status of a given interface. To achieve this, each neuropattern is characterized by the concomitant expression of specific and a priori defined psychological, biological, and symptom variables. If these specific variables are expressed all together, the patient qualifies for a given neuropattern.

4 Lovallo WR, Gerin W: Psychophysiological reactivity: mechanisms and pathways to cardiovascular disease. Psychosom Med 2003;65:36–45.
5 Moran O, Phillip M: Leptin: obesity, diabetes and other peripheral effects – a review. Pediatr Diab 2003;4:101–109.
6 Kaplan MS, Nunes A: The psychosocial determinants of hypertension. Nutr Metab Cardiovasc Dis 2003;13:52–59.
7 Hellhammer DH, Buske-Kirschbaum A: Psychobiologische Aspekte von Schutz und Reparaturenmechanismen; in Lamprecht F, Johnen R (eds): Salutogenese – Ein neues Konzept in der Psychosomatik. Frankfurt-Bockenheim, VAS – Verlag für Akademische Schriften, 1994, pp 95–105.
8 Lazarus RS, Folkman S: Stress, Appraisal and Coping. New York, Springer, 1984.
9 Lacey BC: Somatic response patterning and stress: some revisions of activation theory; in Appley MH, Trumbull R (eds): Psychological Stress: Issues in Research. New York, Appleton-Century-Crofts, 1967.
10 Schlotz W: Kovariation psychoendokriner Stressindikatoren: Analyse von Cortisol und Stresserleben mit Multilevel-Modellen. Berlin, Wissenschaftlicher Verlag Berlin, 2005.
11 Fahrenberg J: Psychophysiologie und Verhaltenstherapie; in Margraf J (ed): Lehrbuch der Verhaltenstherapie, ed 2. Berlin, Springer, 2000, pp 107–124.
12 Herman JP, Prewitt CM, Cullinan WE: Neuronal circuit regulation of the hypothalamo-pituitary-adrenocortical stress axis. Crit Rev Neurobiol 1996;10:371–394.
13 Lopez JF, Akil H, Watson SJ: Neural circuits mediating stress. Biol Psychiatry 1999;46:1461–1471.
14 Pacak K, Palkovits M: Stressor specificity of central neuroendocrine responses: implications for stress-related disorders. Endocr Rev 2001;22:502–548.
15 Charmandari E, Tsigos C, Chrousos G: Endocrinology of the stress response. Ann Rev Physiol 2005;67:259–284.
16 Dallman MF, Pecoraro NC, La Fleur SE, Warne JP, Ginsberg AB, Akana SF, Laugero KC, Houshyar H, Strack AM, Bhatnagar S, Bell ME: Glucocorticoids, chronic stress, and obesity. Prog Brain Res 2006;153:75–105.
17 McEwen BS: Physiology and neurobiology of stress and adaptation: central role of the brain. Physiol Rev 2007;87:873–904.
18 Porges SW: Asserting the role of biobehavioral sciences in translational research: the behavioral neurobiology revolution. Dev Psychopathol 2006;18:923–933.
19 Marincola FM: Translational medicine: a two-way road. J Transl Med 2003;1:1.
20 Schwartz JE, Stone AA: Strategies for analyzing ecological momentary assessment data. Health Psychol 1998;17:6–16.
21 Wittchen H-U, Jacobi F: Psychische Störungen in Deutschland und der EU – Grössenordnung und Belastung. Verhaltensther Psychosoz Praxis 2006;38:189–192.
22 Hoyer J, Helbig S, Wittchen H-U: Experiences with psychotherapy for depression in routine care: a naturalistic patient survey in Germany. Clin Psychol Psychother 2006;13:414–421.
23 Etkin A, Pittenger C, Polan HJ, Kandel ER: Toward a neurobiology of psychotherapy: basic science and clinical applications. J Neuropsychiatry Clin Neurosci 2005;17:145–158.
24 Ellis CR, Singh NN, Landrum TJ: Pharmacotherapy. Part I. J Dev Phys Disab 1993;5:1–4.
25 Kroenke K, Spitzer R: The PHQ9: A new depression diagnostic and severity measure. Psychiatr Annals 2002;32:509–521.
26 Spitzer RL, Kroenke K, Williams JB: Validation and utility of a self-report version of PRIME-MD: the PHQ primary care study. Primary Care Evaluation of Mental Disorders. Patient Health Questionnaire. JAMA 1999;282:1737–1744.
27 Maslach C, Jackson SE, Leiter MP: Maslach Burnout Inventory Manual, ed 3. Palo Alto, Consulting Psychologists Press, 1996.

Hellhammer DH, Hellhammer J (eds): Stress. The Brain-Body Connection.
Key Issues in Mental Health. Basel, Karger, 2008, vol 174, pp 21–38

3. Principles of the Crosstalk between Brain and Body – Glandotropy, Ergotropy, and Trophotropy

Dirk H. Hellhammer

As described in chapter 2, psychobiological processes in humans are tremendously complex, actually still too complex to be described satisfactorily. In a period of continuous growth of knowledge, it turned out to be useful to characterize such processes in terms which make a temporary understanding easier. Examples are psychological terms and constructs such as memory, cognition, emotion, or clinical disorders such as anxiety and depression. If, for example, we talk about the psychobiology of depression, we can quote countless bits of information from the fields of neuroanatomy, neurochemistry, neurophysiology, neuroimaging, genetics, etc. However, if we want to translate this knowledge into clinical practice, or if we try to link it to subjective experiences, we need to be able to use such temporary constructs. In other words, we have to accept meta-level descriptions, implying a good deal of temporary assumptions, when connecting or interpreting the data.

For the brain-body connection, this type of conceptualization was introduced early by the Swiss physiologist and Nobel laureate W.R. Hess [1–3]. Hess chose the terms 'ergotropic' and 'trophotropic' to describe and distinguish the functional roles of the sympathetic and the parasympathetic system as interfaces between psychological processes and bodily responses in adaptation to environmental demands. Following the early terminology of Hess, we now want to use these terms and spread his definitions to the central control mechanisms, which directly modulate the ergotropic and the trophotropic stress response. In addition, we include the hypothalamic-pituitary-adrenal axis (HPAA) as a third (endocrine) system, participating in the crosstalk between the brain and the body. We here refer to the functional role of the HPAA with the term 'glandotropic system' (fig. 3.1.).

It would be misleading to say that the central control mechanisms which we include in this terminology would have only ergotropic, trophotropic, or glandotropic functions. Rather, this characterization refers to only one (major) aspect of these sys-

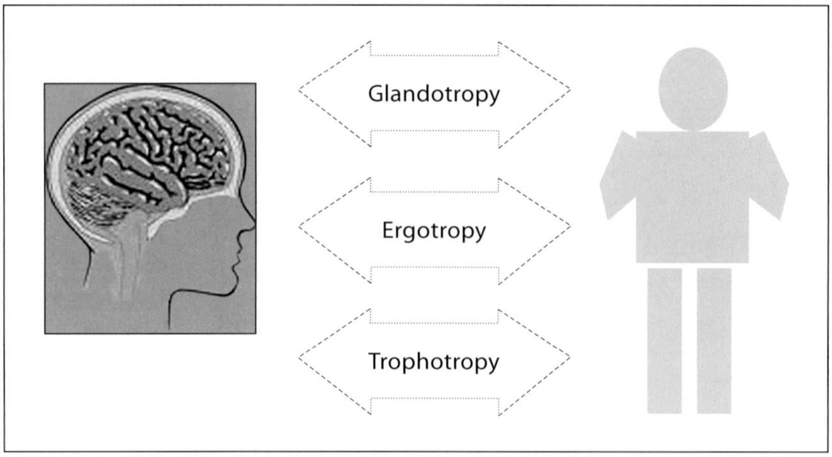

Fig. 3.1. Principles of the crosstalk between brain and body.

tems. In addition, the functions of all three systems are affected by many other systems, which in part act either synergistically or antagonistically. Thus, it would be impossible to precisely narrow down and define these terms neuroanatomically or neurophysiologically. On the other hand, these systems are functionally distinct in their adaptation to stress, and it turned out to be helpful to distinguish them by these terms, particularly for translational purposes.

3.1. Glandotropic Interfaces

In our context, glandotropy refers to the activity of the HPAA in the adaptation to stress. The ability of the organism to exert this glandotropic response is most important to mobilize energy resources by increasing glucose levels, inducing gluconeogenesis, preventing an overshooting of the immune response to stress, increasing blood pressure and facilitating the effectiveness of catecholamines. The glandotropic stress response is delayed with cortisol levels reaching a peak at about 30 min after the onset of the stressor.

The HPAA consists of different parts. The paraventricular nucleus of the hypothalamus (PVN) contains two types of neurons, one secreting corticotropin-releasing factor (CRF) and the other both CRF and arginine vasopressin (AVP). The axons of these neurons project to the median eminence, where they release CRF and AVP into the hypophyseal portal blood vessels, connecting the median eminence with the anterior pituitary. Here, CRF and AVP bind to receptors on cells, which release adrenocorticotropic hormone (ACTH) into the bloodstream. ACTH then stimulates the release of cortisol from the adrenal cortex. Cortisol binds to receptors of numerous target cells in the body, and exerts a negative feedback on the HPAA via receptors in the hippocampus, the PVN and the pituitary [4, 5]. The activity and reactivity status can thus be described at the hypothalamic, pituitary and adrenal level and, in addition, with respect to receptor status. HPAA functions and measures of cortisol can be modified at all these levels. To attempt and estimate a better discrimination, we thus conceptualized several glandotropic neuropatterns.

3.1.1. Paraventricular Nucleus

The activity and reactivity status of the PVN depends on state and trait determinants. Under stress conditions, state determinants comprehend mainly inhibitory effects from glucocorticoid feedback and the hippocampus, and stimulatory effects of the locus coeruleus (LC). Once the hippocampus is active, the paraventricular nucleus becomes activated. This happens if an individual tries to adapt to situations which are perceived as ambiguous, novel, uncontrollable, or unpredictable. In addition, Mason [6] emphasized the importance of 'ego involvement' and anticipation, which both seem to be most relevant if not necessary for psychological stress in activating the HPAA. Anticipatory worrying about uncontrollable, unpredictable, predominantly self-related future events can thus be considered an adequate psychological stimulus for HPAA reactivity [6, 7]. As described in chapter 4, the PVN is able to activate two different subtypes of neurons, probably to allow for adaptation to both acute and chronic stress. The sensitivity of the PVN to respond to these types of stressors or to stimuli from other subsystems of the brain and the body is obviously dependent on genetic and epigenetic determinants (see chapter 4). For diagnostic purposes, it will be helpful to discriminate both activity and reactivity components of PVN activation.

Both, hypoactivity and hyporeactivity of these neurons of the PVN has been proposed to be associated with stress-related disorders. Under these circumstances, the HPAA and the SNS are underactivated and different psychological and somatic symptoms such as listlessness, hypersomnia and weight gain emerge; this is often referred to as 'atypical depression' [8, 9]. In summary, the PVN is an important interface within the brain-body connection, and one could discriminate four states of hyper- and hypoactivity and hyper- and hyporeactivity, respectively.

3.1.2. Anterior Pituitary

The pituitary is not a passive gland, which responds with the linear release of adrenocorticotropin (ACTH) in response to stimulatory input from the PVN [10, 11]. Rather, there are different modulators that finally determine the synthesis of the precursor molecule pro-opiomelanocortin (POMC) and the release of ACTH. The two most important factors are (1) the availability of CRF and AVP receptors, and (2) the degree of inhibitory glucocorticoid feedback [12]. In addition, the expression of POMC is genetically determined [13, 14], and this and pathological conditions may result in a hyper- or hyporeactivity of ACTH release in response to stress.

The release of ACTH from the pituitary is not directly associated with psychological measures, although effects on cognitive performance have been reported [15–17]. With respect to biological measures, the sensitivity of CRF receptors can best be tested by CRF challenge tests [18–20], while the (low-dose) dexamethasone test provides an estimate on glucocorticoid feedback sensitivity, mainly at the pituitary level [21, 22]. These two variables mainly allow assessing ACTH hyper- and hyporeactivity.

Pathological conditions (lesions, tumors) which lead to ACTH deficiency may not only result in low cortisol levels, but also in psychological and somatic symptoms such as fatigue, weakness, nausea, hypotension and weight loss [23, 24]. On the other hand, hypercortisolism (morbus Cushing) is mostly due to ACTH-producing adenomas of the pituitary and promotes hypertension, adipositas, diabetes type 2, osteoporosis, amenorrhea as well as psychiatric symptoms such as major depression mania, anxiety disorders and cognitive dysfunction [25].

As can be seen, it may occasionally be worth screening for characteristic patterns of hyper- and hyposecretion of ACTH, and it may even be possible to differentiate between activity and reactivity measures. Mostly, patterns of ACTH activity will allow a differential diagnosis and treatment of disorders, which have been considered to be stress related. On the other hand, an analysis of hypo- or hyperreactivity of the HPAA to stress needs to consider the role of the pituitary to obtain a correct estimate.

3.1.3. Adrenals

If and how much cortisol is produced by the adrenals depends on different factors. First, the status of the ACTH receptor in the adrenal cortex may be genetically affected [26, 27] or vary with chronic stress [28]. The ability of ACTH to stimulate the release of cortisol from the adrenals can best be assessed by monitoring cortisol levels after administering low doses of synthetic ACTH [29]. However, Synacthen tests cannot be applied easily in the clinical routine. Thus, an assessment of cortisol reactivity is difficult. Considering the pros (increase of information) and cons (Synacthen test), it does not seem worth to include reactivity measures at a first screening procedure.

Since the early work of Hans Selye, it has been known that chronic stress may result in hypercortisolemia, accompanied by enlargement of the adrenal cortex [30]. As described in chapter 4, psychological stressors activate the HPAA via the PVN. Thus, the same psychological characteristics are observed as originally described by Mason [6]. Associated physical symptoms are enhanced blood pressure, abdominal obesity, osteoporosis, diabetes type 2, impaired immune function [31], etc. Indirect effects of impaired glucocorticoid receptor function may further result in a disinhibition of CRF in the PVN, resulting in chronic activation of the HPAA and a similar physical symptomatology (pseudo-Cushing). This mechanism has been considered by Holsboer [32] as a possible cause of major depression. Finally, pathological conditions such as an adrenal adenoma or a carcinoma of the adrenal cortex rarely induce hypercortisolism. Taken together, chronic stress, major depression, and pathological conditions can all result in a gradual hypercortisolism and impair physical health.

However, after prolonged stress, adrenal hyperplasia can persist, although cortisol levels may drop below former baseline levels, thereby manifesting a hypocortisolemic state [33–35]. Thus, both hyper- and hypocortisolism can be observed under chronic stress. The clinical picture of hypocortisolism somewhat resembles Addison's disease [36], with symptoms such as fatigue, weakness, hyperpigmentation, loss in body weight, muscle pain, etc. Today, we believe that hypocortisolemic disorders are most common among stress-related disorders, comprehending a broad array of so-called somatoform disorders, such as chronic fatigue, fibromyalgia, chronic pelvic pain and burnout (see chapter 5) [37].

3.1.4. Glucocorticoid Receptors

Since the HPAA is a homeostatic system, disturbances at the glucocorticoid receptor feedback sites may impair the ability of the HPAA to adapt to stress. This seems true for the central nervous system in facilitating major depression (see above), but also for peripheral glucocorticoid receptors. If the characteristic spectrum of hypocortisolemic symptoms is observed, but cortisol levels are normal, one may assume a deficiency of glucocorticoid receptors on lymphocytes, disabling cortisol to sufficiently inhibit the release of pro-inflammatory cytokines. Under these circumstances, similar hypocortisolemic symptoms, predominantly pain and fatigue, can occur, which have been described as 'sickness behavior' (see chapter 5) [38].

3.2. Ergotropy

The most prominent feature of the acute or immediate stress response is the fight-flight reaction, which was originally described by Cannon [39], and later recognized as the first stage of a general adaptation syndrome [40]. Once a stimulus is perceived as a threat, an intense and prolonged discharge from the LC activates the sympathetic division of the autonomic nervous system [41]. The fight-flight response is predominantly characterized by the release of catecholamines in both the central and the sympathetic nervous systems. Central noradrenergic neurons increase alertness and attention to environmental stimuli and facilitate spontaneous or intuitive behaviors often related to fight or flight. Sympathetic activation triggers increases in heart rate and breathing, constriction of blood vessels, release of glucose and tightening of the muscles. Thus, stressor-induced activation of the LC and the sympathetic nervous system constitute a major component of the brain-body connection.

However, activation of these interfaces is not restricted to the fight-flight response. Hess [1–3] and later many other researchers observed that increased behavioral arousal, cerebral excitation, sympathetic discharges, and somatic effects were not only as-

ment also 'program' noradrenergic hyperreactivity in later life. Evidence for this has been provided in both animals [81, 82] and humans and in the latter such determinants seem to constitute later vulnerability for affective disorders [83].

Under chronic stress, the LC and the synthesis and release of NE is permanently stimulated; if such conditions of chronic stress persist, a depletion of NE storage vesicles will be expected, which can no longer be compensated by a sufficient synthesis of this neurotransmitter, allowing the vesicles to refill [84]. Thus, NE depletion is another scenario which can be observed as a consequence of chronic stress. We here name this state 'NE hyporeactivity', which is characterized by its own specific pattern of psychological, biological, and symptomatic characteristics and which is mainly observed under poststress conditions (see chapter 6).

As the LC is only one (major) player in the ergotropic stress response, others, such as the Ncl. Barrington or the Ncl. tractus solitarius, soon need to be included as important interfaces. However, our psychobiological knowledge is still too fragmentary to include these and other important brain areas which act as ergotropic interfaces within the brain-body connection.

3.2.2. Sympathetic Nervous System

The sympathetic nervous system (SNS) refers to a functional network of preganglionic and postganglionic efferent fibers which innervate tissues and organs throughout the human body with the exception of skeletal muscle fibers. Most postganglionic fibers release NE, with the exception of the adrenal medulla, which mainly releases epinephrine, and, to a lesser extent, NE. Hess [3] described the functions of the SNS as ergotropic, since they synchronize bodily functions for optimal adaptation to fight, flight, or working conditions.

However, functions of the SNS are not only executive to input from the central nervous system, but could be affected by (local) hyper- or hypoactivity/hyper- or hyporeactivity of the gut, the heart, or any other organ. In addition, gene polymorphisms may modulate the efficacy of the catecholamines at receptor sites [69, 85]. This may not only cause interindividual differences in the degree of sympathetically modulated stress responses, but also affect interoception of visceral stimuli, and thus the perceived emotional valence [86–88]. The same may be true, at least in part, for stage fright, where the increase of sympathetic arousal can be prevented well by beta-blockers, while the effects could not be attributed to dampening central arousal [89].

A good clinical example for sympathetic hyperactivity is pheochromocytoma, a catecholamine-producing tumor, which leads not only to peripheral symptoms (headaches, sweating, hypertension, palpitations, etc.), but also to feelings of panic and anxiety [90], since the peripheral events are attributed as dangerous.

On the other hand, a similar picture may emerge in subjects who have (partial) hypoactivity of sympathetic function. Clinical conditions such as diabetes and uremia often develop a peripheral sympathetic neuropathy; heart failure and diseases of the sympathetic nervous system may further result in sympathetic dysfunction. In some patients, both physical and psychological stresses provoke strong sympathetic neuronal responses [91]. Furthermore, lower plasma NE levels have been observed in patients with supine hypertension [92]. As addressed in chapter 6, some patients with low catecholamine levels show enhanced stress responsivity, suggesting a compensatory upregulation of postsynaptic receptor sites.

In summary, to fully understand the ergotropic stress response, it may occasionally be relevant to include assessments of sympathetic reactivity to stress. Hyperresponsive patients may have either a high or a low basal sympathetic tone. To obtain a useful diagnosis, it seems to be necessary to include a careful assessment of peripheral sympathetic arousal. Both the dorsal noradrenergic bundle originating in the LC and the SNS seem to act synergistically in terms of an ergotropic stress response.

3.3. Trophotropy

According to Hess [3], trophotropic responses of the organism protect against overload and allow for regeneration and recovery. Opposite to an ergotropic state, trophotropy is characterized by relaxation, sleepiness and withdrawal from activities. The parasympathetic system extended by part of the serotonergic system in the brain is what we refer to here as trophotropy.

Similar to the dorsal noradrenergic system, serotonergic neurons have their cell bodies in the raphe nuclei of the brain stem. From the dorsal raphe nucleus (DRN), serotonergic neurons project to the basal ganglia, allocortex, neocortex, diencephalon, midbrain and brainstem, and the course of serotonergic neurons is very similar to that of noradrenergic neurons [93, 94].

Given the comparable neuroanatomy of both systems, one may wonder about their functional similarities: Is the serotonergic system likewise a 'cognitive complement of parasympathetic function', and, if so, is there a similar antagonism to noradrenergic and sympathetic functions? These questions are extremely difficult to answer since a lot of the data seem to be paradoxical due to the many specific subsections of this system, multiplicity of receptors, different co-transmitters, numerous interactions, and different methodologies applied in respective research studies.

If we approach the serotonergic system from a trophotropic perspective, its function should meet the following criteria:

(1) Unspecific alterations of serotonergic systems in the brain should generally modulate trophotropic function. This should be seen when serotonergic functions are enhanced or diminished.

If we are interested in general but not specific serotonergic functions, it may be interesting to look at studies on gross manipulations of serotonin (5-HT), preferably in a natural environment. Ellison [95], after applying different treatments, summarized his research findings as follows: '5-HT can be thought of as placing the brain into a state of consciousness appropriate for an animal in his nest (i.e. 5-HT neurons act as relaxers), and as involved in a type of positive affect related to security, whereas NE neurons are dominant when an animal is vigilant, foraging out in the environment to goal-directed approach arousal.' Application of tryptophan, the serotonin precursor which is quickly converted to serotonin in the brain, decreases quarrelsome behavior in humans, and facilitates social dominance in both humans and monkeys. Moskowitz et al. [96, p. 287] regard this as 'behaviors oriented to achieve status and resources'. Further, increasing serotonin availability by either tryptophan or a 5-HT reuptake inhibitor increases affiliative behavior in both species. Selective serotonin reuptake inhibitors (SSRI) have mood enhancing and vitalizing effects. In a review on the subject, Petty et al. [97, p. 11] conclude that 'serotonin is a stabilizing agent, which assists in returning the mind to its homeostatic setpoint.'

On the other hand, a deficit of serotonergic neurotransmission is the most prominent feature of depression. Serotonin deficiency may cause a maladaptive stress response. Indeed, several diseases and disorders have been reported to be associated with low brain serotonin levels, such as depression, violent aggression, premenstrual syndrome, anxiety, obsessive-compulsive behavior and eating disorders [98] (see chapter 7). Under laboratory conditions, serotonin hypoactivity has been studied after dietary tryptophan depletion, and under pharmacological conditions, in knockout mice and patients with obvious evidence of 5-HT deficiency. In healthy volunteers, tryptophan depletion results in a decrease of 5-HT and its metabolite 5-HIAA (5-hydroxy-indol-acetic acid) in the cerebrospinal fluid (CSF). Similar effects on lowering of 5-HT release from serotonergic neurons in virtually all brain regions have been observed in rats. In addition, numerous studies show that effects of tryptophan depletion reverse the antidepressant effects of SSRI [99, 100]. In healthy subjects, moderate psychological effects after acute tryptophan depletion have been reported, such as lowering of mood and memory performance and a moderate increase in impulsivity, aggression, and premenstrual-like symptoms. Interestingly, an improvement in focusing attention has also been reported, which was attributed to the actions of other neurotransmitters, namely acetylcholine. In addition, tryptophan depletion resulted in the expected increase of blood pressure and HPA activity [101, 102].

(2) The serotonergic system should act as a functional counterpart ('brake') of the LC ('accelerator') under stressful conditions.

The dorsal raphe nucleus strongly innervates the LC and exerts its effects predominantly via 5-HT_{1A} receptors. These serotonergic projections to the LC seem to inhibit anxiety, aggression, goal-directed behavior, blood pressure, etc. Interestingly, serotonergic neurons in the raphe nucleus also presynaptically inhibit their own activity via the same receptors, thus decreasing serotonergic neurotransmission in several other brain areas [103, 104]. Tryptophan has also been frequently used as a nonprescription sleep-inducing agent, although the effects of serotonin on sleep are heterogeneous. Obviously, the raphe nucleus can promote slow wave sleep (SWS) via

5-HT_{1A} receptor-mediated effects on the LC [105]. Interestingly, it has recently been shown that a concomitant decrease of SWS and hippocampally mediated memory consolidation occurs. This points to a role of the dorsal raphe nucleus in SWS-modulated memory consolidation, which may be another indicator of trophotropic reconstitutive serotonergic effects [106].

If the effects of the DRN on the LC are enhanced, one may call this 'serotonin hyperactivity', characterized by a stress-dampening effect on both psychological (arousal, aggression, impulsivity, anxiety) and biological variables, such as cardiovascular and HPA activity, while a serotonin deficiency may have the opposite effects and enforce ergotropy [102]. Animal experiments using 5-HT_{1A} receptor knockout mice support this unspecific view of serotonergic function: the animals are more anxious and show elevated body temperature and tachycardia in response to novelty stress. Interestingly, these effects are not as obvious under unstimulated conditions and they seem to habituate under repeated stimulation [107]. This could possibly mean that the stress-buffering effects of serotonin on the LC are related to novelty, unpredictability, and uncontrollability and are mediated by CRF neurons originating in the PVN, which also habituate to stress.

In the autonomic nervous system, the parasympathetic system can buffer overshooting of a sympathetic response. In the brain, both the noradrenergic and the serotonergic systems control their own activity by autoreceptors. In a thorough review, van de Kar and Blair [108, p. 28] conclude that 'the excitatory effect of dorsal raphe projections to the paraventricular nucleus may be mediated by 5-HT_2 or 5-HT_3 receptors. In contrast, 5-HT_{1A} receptor agonists inhibit the effect of psychological stress on renin, prolactin, and corticosterone, possibly by acting on somatodendritic 5-HT_{1A} autoreceptors to reduce the firing rate of dorsal raphe serotonergic neurons.' Thus, presynaptic effects of 5-HT_{1A} receptors may act in a trophotropic manner by preventing an overshooting of the stress response.

(3) Serotonergic functions should act complementary to parasympathetic functions.

The hypothalamus is the major control center of the dorsal nucleus of the vagus (DVN). As reviewed by Palkovits [109], the DVN is bi-directionally connected with the PVN, and these pathways play the central role in the trophotropic adaptation to stress. The PVN controls the DVN via descending peptidergic fibers arising from the ventral medial and lateral parvicellular subdivisons of the PVN. In addition, few additional projections from the arcuate nucleus and the nucleus ambiguus innervate the DVN, while other projections from the lateral hypothalamus (e.g. perifornical and dorsomedial nucleus) control other parasympathetic functions involved in the regulation of fluid homeostasis, body weight, metabolism, feeding, and blood pressure. The role of direct innervations of the DVN from the DR is limited. Wang et al. [110] reported that 5-HT applied to vagal preganglionic neurons evokes both excitatory and inhibitory responses. The excitatory but not the inhibitory responses are likely to be mediated by activation of the 5-HT_{1A} receptors. As mentioned above, 5-HT_{1A} receptor knockout mice did not show autonomic changes under baseline conditions, but emitted an exaggerated response to novelty stress (fearful behavior, tachycardia, hyperthermia), indicating an enhanced fear/anxiety response [107]. Such data refer to the possible (trophotropic) counter-regulation of the stress response, which one can consider physiologically similar to the parasympathetic regulation of autonomic stress responses. This would implicate that such serotonergic neurons are mainly activated under stress. This assumption is met by findings showing an enhanced firing rate and extracellular release of serotonin from dorsal raphe neurons during stress, predominantly at the 5-HT_{1A} receptor sites [111]. Furthermore, neurons from the raphe pallidus and obscurus containing TRH, 5-HT, and substance P project to the dorsal vagal complex DVN. Via the vagus these pathways stimulate gastric secretory and motor function and modulate resistance of the gastric mucosa [112].

(4) Serotonergic functions in the brain should facilitate energy supply and revitalization, particularly under stressful conditions.

Serotonergic effects on the hypothalamus are mostly mediated by 5-HT_2 and 5-HT_3 receptors, and seem to be ergotropic rather than trophotropic in nature [108]. Under adaptation to stress, the brain needs to communicate closely with executive bodily functions. However, the brain itself, as an organ, has other trophotropic requirements. As the parasympathetic system helps the organism to gain new energy by the digestion of food, a trophotropic system in the brain should also assist to guarantee energy supply for the brain. The tool to do so is the activation of the pituitary adrenal axis, e.g. the mobilization of glucose via cortisol release. This mechanism is essential for the brain to regulate its own energy demands under stressful conditions and recovery [59].

In addition, and independent of the stress response, the medial raphe nucleus projects to feeding centers of the brain, where serotonin regulates various downstream neuropeptide systems and autonomic pathways which affect ingestive behavior and energy expenditure. 'Specifically, depletion of brain serotonin promotes hyperphagia (excessive ingestion of food) and obesity, whereas administration of drugs increasing serotonergic transmission, serotonin receptor (5-HTR) agonists and serotonin itself all reduce food intake, decrease body weight and enhance energy expenditure' [113, p. 1]. Thus, the brain may be able to initiate feeding and refilling of energy stores to guarantee intact serotonin function. In some women, a serotonin deficiency in the premenstrual phase is associated with enhanced uptake of carbohydrates. Extensive research by Richard Wurtman's group has shown that carobohydrate consumption enhances the transport of tryptophan into the brain via insulin secretion, and, subsequently, serotonin synthesis and release, facilitating relaxation and enhancing mood and fatigue [114]. Again, it seems that the serotonergic system is able to specifically regulate maintenance of its own trophotropic functions.

Although it seems to be possible to conceptualize serotonergic functions as trophotropic, there are other specific studies which would presently not support such an assumption. Different components of the serotonergic system have different functions, and available knowledge is simply insufficient to fully justify such a conceptualization. In addition, there is currently no method to directly assess 5-HT synaptic levels in living human brains [115]. Thus, it is difficult to concretely characterize and specify trophotropic serotonergic functions in humans. This would be helpful and ultimately necessary to generalize data from animal experiments, particularly facing species differences in neuronal subtypes, receptors and functions [115–117].

3.3.1. Parasympathetic Nervous System

Many stress-related symptoms are parasympathetically mediated. Examples are gastrointestinal, cardiac and pulmonary disorders. The different efferent branches of the parasympathetic system (PNS), especially the vagus, can vary both interindividually and regionally in terms of basal activity and reactivity. Thus, it seems to be important to assess such variables in diagnostic treatments in stress medicine separately.

As the trophotropic counterpart of the SNS, the PNS activates gastrointestinal function, thus allowing digestion and refilling of energy reservoirs. The PNS dampens heart frequency, blood pressure and pulmonary function in phases of rest, facilitating regeneration and preserving organ function [118]. There is a wide range of parasympathetically mediated symptoms, which typically occur after stress exposure or under conservation withdrawal behavior, such as bradycardia, hypotonia, gastrointestinal complaints, asthma, or myalgia. In chapter 7, we address different disorders, which are biased by parasympathetic hyper- and hypoactivity and hyper- and hyporeactivity. Notably, all these traits and states are results of the interplay between the SNS and the PNS.

From an integrated psychobiological and phylogenetic viewpoint, Porges [119] conceptualized the role of the vagus as an adaptive system to environmental demands. His 'polyvagal theory' considers CNS–ANS interactions and discriminates three ANS components: (1) the unmyelinated vagus (or dorsal vagal complex), which mediates immobility and passive avoidance; (2) the sympathetic-adrenal system, which mobilizes the organism and active avoidance, and (3) the myelinated vagus or ventral vagal complex, which participates in social communication, self-soothing, calming and inhibiting arousal: 'Functionally, when the environment is perceived as safe, two important features are expressed. First, the bodily state is regulated in an efficient manner to promote growth and restoration (e.g. visceral homeostasis). This is done through an increase in the influence of myelinated vagal motor pathways on the cardiac pacemaker that slows the heart, inhibits the fight/flight mechanisms of the sympathetic nervous system, dampens the stress response system of the HPA-axis (e.g. cortisol), and reduces inflammation by modulating immune reactions (e.g. cytokines). Second, through the process of evolution, the brainstem nuclei that regulate the myelinated vagus became integrated with the nuclei that regulate the muscles of the face and head. This link results in the bi-directional coupling between spontaneous social engagement behaviors and bodily states' [119, p. 120].

It should be noted that serotonergic and parasympathetic functions vary with the impact of genetic and developmental factors, which is addressed specifically in chapter 7. Taken together, this brief overview illustrates that it seems reasonable to focus on both the dorsal raphe nucleus and the parasympathetic system as functionally diverse inferfaces of the brain-body connection. Stress-related parasympathetic dysfunction seems to predominantly occur in consequence of NE depletion. A hyperserotonergic state, on the other hand, may primarily buffer an ergotropic stress response, and only rarely be of clinical significance itself.

In summary, the response to acute and chronic stress varies with the activity and reactivity of the raphe nuclei. The DR is particularly important by buffering the ergotropic stress response and affecting the outflow of HPAA and ANS. The functions are associated with discrete changes in psychological, biological, and symptom measures, depending from the respective (re-)activity status.

3.4. Summary

To facilitate the translation of basic research findings to clinical application, we conceptualized the principles of the crosstalk between brain and body, which constitute the stress response. While 'glandotropy' mainly refers to the pituitary-adrenal-axis, the traditional terms 'ergotropy' and 'trophotropy' refer to the autonomic nervous system. They were extended to the biogenic amine systems, which are functionally associated with the HPAA and ANS.

References

1 Hess WR: Über die Wechselbeziehungen zwischen psychischen und vegetativen Funktionen. Schweiz Arch Neurol Psychiatr 1924;15:260–277.
2 Hess WR: Ueber die Wechselbeziehungen zwischen psychischen und vegetativen Funktionen. Schweiz Arch Neurol Psychiatr 1925;16:36–55.
3 Hess WR: Die physiologischen Grundlagen der Psychosomatik. Dtsch Med Wochenschr 1961;86: 3–8.
4 Kirschbaum C, Hellhammer DH: Hypothalamus-Hypophysen-Nebennierenrindenachse; in Hellhammer DH, Kirschbaum C (eds): Enzyklopädie der Psychologie, Psychoendokrinologie und Psychoimmunologie. Biologische Psychologie. Göttingen, Hogrefe, 1999, pp 79–140.
5 Ganong WF, Dallman MF, Roberts JL: The Hypothalamic-Pituitary-Adrenal Axis Revisited: A Symposium in Honor of Dorothy Krieger and Edward Herbert. New York, New York Academy of Sciences, 1987.
6 Mason JW: A review of psychoendocrine research on the pituitary-adrenal cortical system. Psychosom Med 1968;30:576–607.
7 Hellhammer DH: Gehirn und Verhalten. Eine anwendungsorientierte Einführung in die Psychobiologie. Münster, Aschendorff, 1983.
8 Gold PW, Chrousos GP: Organization of the stress system and its dysregulation in melancholic and atypical depression: high vs. low CRH/NE states. Mol Psychiatry 2002;7:254–275.
9 Rapaport MH, Thase ME: Translating the evidence on atypical depression into clinical practice. J Clin Psychiatry 2007;68:e11.

10 Aguilera G, Nikodemova M, Wynn PC, Catt KJ: Corticotropin releasing hormone receptors: two decades later. Peptides 2004;25:319–329.
11 Watts AG: Glucocorticoid regulation of peptide genes in neuroendocrine CRH neurons: a complexity beyond negative feedback. Front Neuroendocrinol 2005;26:109–130.
12 Murakami I, Takeuchi S, Kudo T, Sutou S, Takahashi S: Corticotropin-releasing hormone or dexamethasone regulates rat pro-opiomelanocortin transcription through Tpit/Pitx-responsive element in its promoter. J Endocrinol 2007;193:279–290.
13 Chen Y, Snieder H, Wang X, Kaviya B, McCaffrey C, Spector TD, Carter ND, O'Dell SD: Proopiomelanocortin gene variants are associated with serum leptin and body fat in a normal female population. Eur J Hum Genet 2005;13:772–780.
14 Sutton BS, Langefeld CD, Williams AH, Norris JM, Saad MF, Haffner SM, Bowden DW: Association of proopiomelanocortin gene polymorphisms with obesity in the IRAS family study. Obes Res 2005;13:1491–1498.
15 de Wied D, van Ree JM: Neuropeptides, mental performance and aging. Life Sci 1982;31:709–719.
16 Greven HM, de Wied D: The influence of peptides derived from corticotrophin (ACTH) on performance: structure activity studies. Prog Brain Res 1973;39:429–442.
17 Fehm-Wolfsdorf G, Elbert T, Lutzenberger W, Rockstroh B, Birbaumer N, Fehm HL: Effect of an ACTH 4–9 analog on human cortical evoked potentials in a two-stimulus reaction time paradigm. Psychoneuroendocrinology 1981;6:311–320.
18 Gold PW, Chrousos G, Kellner C, Post R, Roy A, Augerinos P, Schulte H, Oldfield E, Loriaux DL: Psychiatric implications of basic and clinical studies with corticotropin-releasing factor. Am J Psychiatry 1984;141:619–627.
19 Holsboer F, Gerken A, Stalla GK, Muller OA: ACTH, cortisol, and corticosterone output after ovine corticotropin-releasing factor challenge during depression and after recovery. Biol Psychiatry 1985;20:276–286.
20 Heuser I, Yassouridis A, Holsboer F: The combined dexamethasone/CRH test: a refined laboratory test for psychiatric disorders. J Psychiatr Res 1994;28:341–356.
21 de Kloet CS, Vermetten E, Geuze E, Kavelaars A, Heijnen CJ, Westenberg HG: Assessment of HPA-axis function in posttraumatic stress disorder: pharmacological and non-pharmacological challenge tests, a review. J Psychiatr Res 2006;40:550–567.
22 Kalin NH, Risch SC, Janowsky DS, Murphy DL: Use of dexamethasone suppression test in clinical psychiatry. J Clin Psychopharmacol 1981;1:64–69.
23 Klose M, Watt T, Brennum J, Feldt-Rasmussen U: Posttraumatic hypopituitarism is associated with an unfavorable body composition and lipid profile, and decreased quality of life 12 months after injury. J Clin Endocrinol Metab 2007;92:3861–3868.
24 Sheppard M, Stewart P: Pituitary Diseases, ed 1. Norwell, Kluwer Academic Publishers, 2002.
25 Sonino N, Fava GA: Psychiatric disorders associated with Cushing's syndrome: epidemiology, pathophysiology and treatment. CNS Drugs 2001;15:361–373.
26 Metherell LA, Chapple JP, Cooray S, David A, Becker C, Ruschendorf F, Naville D, Begeot M, Khoo B, Nurnberg P, Huebner A, Cheetham ME, Clark AJ: Mutations in MRAP, encoding a new interacting partner of the ACTH receptor, cause familial glucocorticoid deficiency type 2. Nat Genet 2005;37:166–170.
27 Slawik M, Reisch N, Zwermann O, Maser-Gluth C, Stahl M, Klink A, Reincke M, Beuschlein F: Characterization of an adrenocorticotropin (ACTH) receptor promoter polymorphism leading to decreased adrenal responsiveness to ACTH. J Clin Endocrinol Metab 2004;89:3131–3137.
28 Aguilera G, Kiss A, Lu A, Camacho C: Regulation of adrenal steroidogenesis during chronic stress. Endocr Res 1996;22:433–443.
29 Schmidt-Reinwald A, Pruessner JC, Hellhammer DH, Federenko I, Rohleder N, Schurmeyer TH, Kirschbaum C: The cortisol response to awakening in relation to different challenge tests and a 12-hour cortisol rhythm. Life Sci 1999;64:1653–1660.
30 Selye H: Endocrine reactions during stress. Curr Res Anesth Analg 1956;35:182–193.
31 Chrousos GP, Kino T: Glucocorticoid action networks and complex psychiatric and/or somatic disorders. Stress 2007;10:213–219.
32 Holsboer F: The corticosteroid receptor hypothesis of depression. Neuropsychopharmacology 2000;23:477–501.
33 Hellhammer DH, Wade S: Endocrine correlates of stress vulnerability. Psychother Psychosom 1993;60:8–17.
34 Reber SO, Birkeneder L, Veenema AH, Obermeier F, Falk W, Straub RH, Neumann ID: Adrenal insufficiency and colonic inflammation after a novel chronic psycho-social stress paradigm in mice: implications and mechanisms. Endocrinology 2007;148:670–682.
35 Reber SO, Obermeier F, Straub RH, Falk W, Neumann ID: Chronic intermittent psychosocial stress (social defeat/overcrowding) in mice increases the severity of an acute DSS-induced colitis and impairs regeneration. Endocrinology 2006;147:4968–4976.
36 Nieman LK, Chanco Turner ML: Addison's disease. Clin Dermatol 2006;24:276–280.

37 Heim C, Ehlert U, Hellhammer DH: The potential role of hypocortisolism in the pathophysiology of stress-related bodily disorders. Psychoneuroendocrinology 2000;25:1–35.
38 Dantzer R: Cytokine, sickness behavior, and depression. Neurol Clin 2006;24:441–460.
39 Cannon WB: The emergency function of the adrenal medulla in pain and the major emotions. Am J Physiol 1914;33:356–372.
40 Selye H: Perspectives in stress research. Perspect Biol Med 1959;2:403–416.
41 Thase ME, Howland RH: Biological processes in depression: an updated review and integration; in Beckham EE, Leber WR (eds): Handbook of Depression: Treatment, Assessment, and Research. Homewood, Dorsey Press, 1985.
42 Janig W, Baron R: Complex regional pain syndrome: mystery explained? Lancet Neurol 2003;2: 687–697.
43 Gellhorn E: The emotions and the ergotropic and trophotropic systems. Psychol Forsch 1970;34:48–94.
44 Stahl SM: Essential Psychopharmacology. New York, Cambridge University Press, 2002.
45 Carelli RM: Nucleus accumbens cell firing and rapid dopamine signaling during goal-directed behaviors in rats. Neuropharmacology 2004;47(suppl 1):180–189.
46 Di Chiara G, Bassareo V, Fenu S, De Luca MA, Spina L, Cadoni C, Acquas E, Carboni E, Valentini V, Lecca D: Dopamine and drug addiction: the nucleus accumbens shell connection. Neuropharmacology 2004;47(suppl 1):227–241.
47 Self DW: Regulation of drug-taking and -seeking behaviors by neuroadaptations in the mesolimbic dopamine system. Neuropharmacology 2004;47 (suppl 1):242–255.
48 Van Bockstaele EJ, Aston-Jones G: Integration in the ventral medulla and coordination of sympathetic, pain and arousal functions. Clin Exp Hypertens 1995;17:153–165.
49 Valentino RJ, Aston-Jones GS: Physiological and Anatomical Determinants of Locus Coeruleus Discharge; in Bloom F, Kupfer D (eds): Psychopharmacology: The Fourth Generation of Progress. New York, Raven Press, 1995, pp 373–385.
50 James W: What is an emotion? Mind 1884;9:188–205.
51 James W: Physical basis of emotion. Psychol Rev 1894;101:205–210.
52 Lange C: Ueber Gemüthsbewegungen: Eine psycho-physiologische Studie; in Rand B (ed): The Classical Psychologists. Boston, Houghton Mifflin, 1887, pp 672–684.
53 Dishman RK, Renner KJ, White-Welkley JE, Burke KA, Bunnell BN: Treadmill exercise training augments brain norepinephrine response to familiar and novel stress. Brain Res Bull 2000;52:337–342.
54 Charmandari E, Tsigos C, Chrousos G: Endocrinology of the stress response. Ann Rev Physiol 2005;67:259–284.
55 Dallman MF, Akana SF, Strack AM, Scribner KS, Pecoraro N, La Fleur SE, Houshyar H, Gomez F: Chronic stress-induced effects of corticosterone on brain: direct and indirect. Ann NY Acad Sci 2004; 1018:141–150.
56 Pavcovich LA, Valentino RJ: Regulation of a putative neurotransmitter effect of corticotropin-releasing factor: effects of adrenalectomy. J Neurosci 1997;17:401–408.
57 Schommer NC, Hellhammer DH, Kirschbaum C: Dissociation between reactivity of the hypothalamus-pituitary-adrenal axis and the sympathetic-adrenal-medullary system to repeated psychosocial stress. Psychosom Med 2003;65:450–460.
58 Foote S, Aston-Jones G: Pharmacology and physiology of central noradrenergic systems; in Bloom F, Kupfer DJ (eds): Psychopharmacology: The Fourth Generation of Progress. New York, Raven Press, 1995, pp 335–345.
59 Fehm HL, Kern W, Peters A: The selfish brain: competition for energy resources. Prog Brain Res 2006;153:129–140.
60 Guyenet PG: The sympathetic control of blood pressure. Nat Rev 2006;7:335–346.
61 Kuo LE, Kitlinska JB, Tilan JU, Li L, Baker SB, Johnson MD, Lee EW, Burnett MS, Fricke ST, Kvetnansky R, Herzog H, Zukowska Z: Neuropeptide Y acts directly in the periphery on fat tissue and mediates stress-induced obesity and metabolic syndrome. Nat Med 2007;13:803–811.
62 Kalia M: Neurobiology of sleep. Metabolism: clinical and experimental. 2006;55(10 suppl 2):S2–S6.
63 Pertovaara A: Noradrenergic pain modulation. Prog Neurobiol 2006;80:53–83.
64 Charney SD, Bremner JD, Redmond DE Jr: Noradrenergic neural substrates for anxiety and fear: clinical associations based on preclinical research; in Bloom F, Kupfer DJ (eds): Psychopharmacology: The Fourth Generation of Progress. New York, Raven Press, 1995, pp 387–395.
65 Raskind MA, Peskind ER, Hoff DJ, Hart KL, Holmes HA, Warren D, Shofer J, O'Connell J, Taylor F, Gross C, Rohde K, McFall ME: A parallel group placebo controlled study of prazosin for trauma nightmares and sleep disturbance in combat veterans with post-traumatic stress disorder. Biol Psychiatry 2007;61:928–934.

66 Strawn JR, Geracioti TD Jr: Noradrenergic dysfunction and the psychopharmacology of posttraumatic stress disorder. Depress Anxiety 2007;Mar 12:[Epub ahead of print].
67 Esler M, Alvarenga M, Pier C, Richards J, El-Osta A, Barton D, Haikerwal D, Kaye D, Schlaich M, Guo L, Jennings G, Socratous F, Lambert G: The neuronal noradrenaline transporter, anxiety and cardiovascular disease. J Psychopharmacol (Oxford) 2006;20(4 suppl):60–66.
68 Holmes A, le Guisquet AM, Vogel E, Millstein RA, Leman S, Belzung C: Early life genetic, epigenetic and environmental factors shaping emotionality in rodents. Neurosci Biobehav Rev 2005;29:1335–1346.
69 Jabbi M, Kema IP, van der Pompe G, te Meerman GJ, Ormel J, den Boer JA: Catechol-o-methyltransferase polymorphism and susceptibility to major depressive disorder modulates psychological stress response. Psychiatr Genet 2007;17:183–193.
70 Kirstein SL, Insel PA: Autonomic nervous system pharmacogenomics: a progress report. Pharmacol Rev 2004;56:31–52.
71 Ressler KJ, Nemeroff CB: Role of norepinephrine in the pathophysiology and treatment of mood disorders. Biol Psychiatry 1999;46:1219–1233.
72 Hellhammer DH: Psychobiologische Ansätze bei der Anorexia nervosa; in Meermann R (ed): Anorexia nervosa – Ursachen und Behandlung. Stuttgart, Enke, 1981, pp 43–55.
73 Kaye WH, Ebert MH, Raleigh M, Lake R: Abnormalities in CNS monoamine metabolism in anorexia nervosa. Arch Gen Psychiatry 1984;41:350–355.
74 Soldani P, Fornai F: The functional anatomy of noradrenergic neurons in Parkinson's disease. Funct Neurol 1999;14:97–109.
75 Mann DM, Yates PO: Neurotransmitter deficits in Alzheimer's disease and in other dementing disorders. Hum Neurobiol 1986;5:147–158.
76 Cubells JF, Zabetian CP: Human genetics of plasma dopamine beta-hydroxylase activity: applications to research in psychiatry and neurology. Psychopharmacology 2004;174:463–476.
77 Paladini CA, Beckstead MJ, Weinshenker D: Electrophysiological properties of catecholaminergic neurons in the norepinephrine-deficient mouse. Neuroscience 2007;144:1067–1074.
78 Weinshenker D, Miller NS, Blizinsky K, Laughlin ML, Palmiter RD: Mice with chronic norepinephrine deficiency resemble amphetamine-sensitized animals. Proc Natl Acad Sci USA 2002;99:13873–13877.
79 Schmidt ED, Schoffelmeer AN, De Vries TJ, Wardeh G, Dogterom G, Bol JG, Binnekade R, Tilders FJ: A single administration of interleukin-1 or amphetamine induces long-lasting increases in evoked noradrenaline release in the hypothalamus and sensitization of ACTH and corticosterone responses in rats. Eur J Neurosci 2001;13:1923–1930.
80 Bremner JD, Krystal JH, Southwick SM, Charney DS: Noradrenergic mechanisms in stress and anxiety. I. Preclinical studies. Synapse 1996;23:28–38.
81 Caldji C, Tannenbaum B, Sharma S, Francis D, Plotsky PM, Meaney MJ: Maternal care during infancy regulates the development of neural systems mediating the expression of fearfulness in the rat. Proc Natl Acad Sci USA 1998;95:5335–5340.
82 Liu D, Caldji C, Sharma S, Plotsky PM, Meaney MJ: Influence of neonatal rearing conditions on stress-induced adrenocorticotropin responses and norepinephrine release in the hypothalamic paraventricular nucleus. J Neuroendocrinol 2000;12:5–12.
83 Heim C, Nemeroff CB: The role of childhood trauma in the neurobiology of mood and anxiety disorders: preclinical and clinical studies. Biol Psychiatry 2001;49:1023–1039.
84 Finlay JM, Zigmond MJ, Abercrombie ED: Increased dopamine and norepinephrine release in medial prefrontal cortex induced by acute and chronic stress: effects of diazepam. Neuroscience 1995;64:619–628.
85 Mandelli L, Serretti A, Marino E, Pirovano A, Calati R, Colombo C: Interaction between serotonin transporter gene, catechol-O-methyltransferase gene and stressful life events in mood disorders. Int J Neuropsychopharmacol 2007;10:437–447.
86 Craig AD: Human feelings: why are some more aware than others? Trends Cogn Sci 2004;8:239–241.
87 Dunn BD, Dalgleish T, Lawrence AD: The somatic marker hypothesis: a critical evaluation. Neurosci Biobehav Rev 2006;30:239–271.
88 Pollatos O, Herbert BM, Matthias E, Schandry R: Heart rate response after emotional picture presentation is modulated by interoceptive awareness. Int J Psychophysiol 2007;63:117–124.
89 Brantigan CO, Brantigan TA, Joseph N: Effect of beta blockade and beta stimulation on stage fright. Am J Med 1982;72:88–94.
90 Zelinka T, Eisenhofer G, Pacak K: Pheochromocytoma as a catecholamine producing tumor: implications for clinical practice. Stress 2007;10:195–203.
91 Ziegler MG, Ruiz-Ramon P, Shapiro MH: Abnormal stress responses in patients with diseases affecting the sympathetic nervous system. Psychosom Med 1993;55:339–346.
92 Goldstein DS, Pechnik S, Holmes C, Eldadah B, Sharabi Y: Association between supine hypertension and orthostatic hypotension in autonomic failure. Hypertension 2003;42:136–142.
93 Azmitia EC, Segal M: An autoradiographic analysis of the differential ascending projections of the dorsal and median raphe nuclei in the rat. J Comp Neurol 1978;179:641–667.

4.1.1. Genetically Determined HPAA Hyperactivity

At least four polymorphisms of the glucocorticoid receptor type II (GR) impacting on glucocorticoid sensitivity and different metabolic parameters are currently being investigated. The N363S single nucleotide polymorphism, a point mutation in the codon 363 of exon 2, which changes the codon from asparagine to serine [8], was associated with hypercortisolism and a reduced GR number per cell in an elderly Dutch cohort. Furthermore, heterozygous carriers of this mutation (n = 13 of a total sample of 216 subjects) displayed significantly stronger cortisol suppression in reaction to a low-dose dexamethasone suppression test, increased sensitivity to exogenous glucocorticoids, increased insulin response to dexamethasone, and a higher BMI [9, 10]. Further investigation in different populations revealed an inconsistent picture, however: no associations with BMI, waist-to-hip ratio or glucocorticoid sensitivity were reported, while other studies were in line with the above findings (for review, see [11]). Interestingly, a study investigating acute responses to psychosocial laboratory stress in healthy young males found significantly increased salivary cortisol responses in carriers, suggesting HPAA hyperreactivity in these subjects [12].

The restriction fragment length polymorphism *Bcl*I, identified by Murray et al. [13], consists of a short and a long fragment due to a C→G mutation. In homozygous GG carriers, Panarelli et al. [14] reported increased skin vasoconstriction after glucocorticoid administration; however, glucocorticoid sensitivity in leukocytes tended to be lower. Furthermore, carriers had a tendency towards higher cortisol levels in the morning. An association between this polymorphism and different components of the metabolic syndrome is being discussed.

Another RFLP, named *Tth111*I, residing in the promoter region and first described by Detera-Wadleigh et al. [15], was associated with altered diurnal cortisol regulation, as found in a study by Rosmond et al. [16]. In this study, cortisol secretion was 30–40% higher in homozygous carriers of the long allele, with particularly high values in the evening. There were, however, no differences between carriers and noncarriers in response to dexamethasone, a test meal or metabolic parameters.

Fourthly, lower cholesterol and fasting insulin concentrations and a lower cortisol suppression after 1 mg dexamethasone premedication was found in carriers of the combined point mutation ER22/23EK, indicating relative glucocorticoid resistance (for review, see [11]). The *Bcl*I and ER22/23EK polymorphisms were further found to be associated with a higher susceptibility to develop major depression [17].

4.1.2. Epigenetically Determined HPAA Hyperactivity

It has long been known that early life adversities may influence behavior and HPAA functioning in a long-term fashion [18, 19]. To date, a host of studies report an association between early life components and mental or physical disorders in adulthood in such disorders which may be mediated by alterations in stress system functioning (for reviews, see [20–22]). The common hypothesis underlying such research is that unfavorable prenatal or early postnatal events may alter central nervous system functions critical for the regulation of stress reactions. In the long run and, possibly, only after secondary severe stress challenge, this may contribute to the development of stress-related disorders [23–26]. It is believed that during the phase of early brain maturation, alterations in the epigenome may be the critical factor underlying programming effects.

In an exciting series of studies, Meaney and co-workers were able to trace back effects of early life stress down to the (epi)genetic level [27, 28]. They used rat dams especially bred for displaying extremities of naturally occurring rodent care behavior, thus having a group of dams providing high care to their offspring as operationalized by high frequencies of pup licking and grooming and arch-back nursing versus dams exhibiting low care. In accordance with the dam's behavior, pups developed conspicuous stress-related features in adulthood: rats formerly reared by low-care dams had higher HPA reactions to stress, higher diurnal corticosterone peak levels and showed higher anxiety compared to pups reared by high-care dams. Remarkably, these disparities met an analogue at the molecular level in a CNS structure critical for HPAA regulation, the hippocampus. Meaney et al. were able to show that depending on these neonatal environmental influences, GR protein expression and the underlying epigenetic architecture of the GR gene was altered in adult animals: while CpG methylation within the NGFI-A transcription factor binding site in the GR promoter region was always evident in adult offspring reared by low-caring dams, this site was only rarely methylated in offspring from high-caring dams. As a consequence, offspring of high-caring dams expressed a significantly higher amount of hippocampal GR than offspring from low-caring dams. The hippocampus is considered a major inhibitory HPAA feedback site under stress conditions [29]. Thus, alterations in its functioning may considerably impact on HPAA reactivity to stressors. Additionally, the pattern of methylation remained constant until adulthood, but could only be induced within a subtle time window, i.e. in this case, during the first week of life. Epigenetic processes may therefore functionally explain persisting behavioral and endocrine alterations in subjects who underwent adversities in an early phase of life. However, the exact time window crucial to such effects in other species, and, in particular, in humans, still remains a matter of debate.

4.1.3. Acquired HPAA Hyperactivity

Major critical life events, chronic stress and other conditions coinciding with HPA hyperactivity may elicit the development of stress-related disorders [30–33]. It is assumed that within a phase of prolonged HPA hyperactivation, sensitization of brain pathways may occur, potentially resulting in chronic HPA hyperactivity. However, these processes, to date, are not yet entirely understood (see section 4.2.2. for details).

4.1.4. Interaction of All Three Factors

Which role does each of these factors play in the etiopathology of stress-related disorders? Is one factor sufficient? Or do we rather expect interactions consistent with a diathesis stress model? In terms of pre- and postnatal stress factors, one can argue that such adversities per se may predispose to later morbidity, but effects are most pronounced when later paired with further traumatization. A study by Heim et al. [34] tried to sort out these questions with regard to the development of depression using a multiple linear regression approach in a sample of 49 women. This group consisted of women reporting abuse in early childhood with/without current depression, depressed women without early abuse, and a healthy control group. The outcome measures were plasma ACTH and cortisol reactions to laboratory psychosocial stress. ACTH reactions could be explained by the interaction of early abuse and later trauma in adulthood. Early abuse per se contributed to increased ACTH responsiveness, while reactions were further enhanced with additional traumatization in adulthood. Interestingly, cortisol output could not be significantly predicted, which may indicate a greater adaptive range at the adrenal level.

A longitudinal study on depression in children and adolescents concluded that adverse prenatal influences operationalized as low birth weight were a significant predictor of adolescent depression in girls per se, and furthermore strongly increased the vulnerability to develop depressive symptoms with additional traumatization in childhood and adolescence. According to the authors' findings, prenatal stress constitutes a general susceptibility for the later development of stress disorders, which is fundamentally more incisive than adversities occurring at a later stage in life [35].

4.2. Chronic Stress Exposure, HPA Sensitization and Stress Disorders

The acute response to stress enables the organism to adequately react to threat. Central nervous system functions are biased towards increased stressor-related vigilance, while blood glucose levels and cardiac tone are increased, and systems noncritical to acute survival such as reproduction, feeding and growth are inhibited [7, 36, 37].

Interestingly, two stressor entities can be differentiated, i.e. stressors which require cognitive processing and evaluating, such as establishing a social hierarchy or, in animals, restraint stress, and, on the other hand, a subset of stressors, which is largely physiological, such as hypoxia or volume loss. Only stressors of the first group seem to engage the limbic system, with its prominent components, the hippocampus and the amygdala, and, furthermore, the prefrontal cortex. Stressors of the latter group activate brain stem pathways and the paraventricular nucleus (PVN) to quickly and efficiently initiate compensative reactions in order to prevent life-threatening physiological states such as acute lack of oxygen. In terms of human stress research, we are mainly interested in chronic alterations in the limbic pathways and their interplay with emotion and cognition.

A CNS structure linking both important branches of the endocrine stress system, i.e. the HPAA and the sympathetic-adrenal medullary system, appears to be the locus coeruleus (LC). A set of CRF-containing neurons originating in the PVN, but different from those leading down to the median eminence, send projections to brainstem noradrenergic neurons, among others, to the peri-LC region, into which dendrites of the LC largely extend [38, 39]. Due to its large network of neurons containing the neurotransmitter norepinephrine (NE) that project to a host of cortical and subcortical structures and might therefore synchronize brain activity, the LC is a nucleus critical to attention and arousal processes [7, 40].

Reciprocal pathways exist between the paraventricular CRF system and the LC/NE system [7, 41], though influences do not seem to be equal: activation of the PVN via LC stimulation seems to be stronger and quicker than vice versa, suggesting indirect activation [42], perhaps via the dorsomedial nucleus. Also, CRF-containing neurons originating in the central nucleus of the amygdala (CeA) are part of these projections [40]. Activation of the LC/NE system recruits the sympathetic nervous system (see chapters 3, 6), further inhibiting autonomic vegetative systems and functions, such as feeding or sleep [43].

4.2.1. Shut-Down of HPA Activity

Cortisol dose-dependently inhibits HPA activity via binding to glucocorticoid receptors at the hippocampal and pituitary level, while other sites and mechanisms of inhibitory glucocorticoid feedback are still subject of discussion. The classic concept of glucocorticoid feedback action is that glucocorticoids, after passively diffusing into the cell, bind to their intracellular receptors and cause translocation to the nucleus and consequent alterations at the genomic level. However, sufficient evidence points towards another fast, nongenomic inhibitory action of glucocorticoids, which may involve actions on membrane receptors [29, 44–49]. Interestingly, glucocorticoid inhibition appears to have specific properties according to the type of stressor [50].

4.2.2. Sensitization

Responses to acute stressors are generally considered to be adaptive. On the contrary, chronic stress exposure may result in the development of cardiovascular disease, infertility, or depressive episodes with suicidal tendencies, which all threat survival of the individual and the collective [51, 52]. Doesn't one get used to repeated stressors?

In animal experiments, chronic stress exposure has been shown to cause sensitization of HPAA responses to novel stress. Whereas the repeated exposure to the same source of stress normally leads to habituation in animals and humans, i.e. lower glucocorticoid output with repeated exposures in chronically stressed animals, exposure to a novel stressor eventually causes higher stress hormone responses than in control animals [53, 54]. Furthermore, the autonomic response to repeated homotypic stress does not seem to underlie habituation, but remains relatively constant over exposure trials [53].

Long-lasting alterations in nonhypothalamic CRF pathways are discussed as physiological correlates of sensitization. In particular, increased CRF activity within the

CeA is suspected to play a critical role in mediating shifts in behavioral, neuroendocrine and metabolic functions observed as a consequence of glucocorticoid hypersecretion [7, 55–58]. It has been shown that chronic or intense acute stress, as well as glucocorticoid administration, upregulates CRF expression in the CeA and bed nucleus of the stria terminalis (BNST) in rodents [59–61]. The amygdala is a key structure for linking emotional aspects to experience. Especially its participation in the fear response and anxiety has been the focus of extensive research [62, 63]. The application of a CRF receptor antagonist into the CeA, for example, reduces stress-dependent anxiety, as observed in rats [64, 65]. Elevations in CRF levels, particularly in the CeA, might thus have a considerable impact on psychological parameters such as anxiety, worrying and stress sensitivity.

The CeA sends CRFergic projections to the n. parabrachialis and the BNST, with the latter being connected to the n. dorsalis vagus and, again, the n. parabrachialis. Stimulating those projections to the n. parabrachialis has been shown to elicit shortness of breath and dyspnea. Stimulating afferents heading towards the n. dorsalis vagus may cause bradycardia, an urge to urinate/defecate, while furthermore promoting ulcerations in the upper digestive tract. Due to these relations, one can speculate that such autonomic dysfunctions may coincide with hypercortisolism, whereas in hypocortisolism, an imbalance favoring sympathetic activity should rather be expected [7].

Furthermore, glucocorticoid hypersecretion upregulates CRF expression within the small subset of paraventricular CRF neurons leading to the LC. This mechanism links HPAA activity to sympathetic tone and is discussed in explaining stress-like symptoms in melancholic depression [7, 42]. Further, in animals, chronic stress is associated with a higher secretion of arginine-vasopressin (AVP) colocalized with CRF in a different subset of paraventricular neurons [39, 66]. AVP potentiates actions of CRF and thus enhances ACTH secretion [67]. Interestingly, AVP-induced ACTH release is also less sensitive to the inhibitory actions of glucocorticoids at the pituitary level [66, 68]. Additionally, massive stimulation of the adrenals with ACTH results in adrenal hypertrophy and elevated glucocorticoid output [69].

Another peripheral mechanism affecting glucocorticoid availability refers to the main glucocorticoid carrier protein, cortisol-binding globulin (CBG). According to the free hormone concept [70], only the unbound glucocorticoid fraction is biologically active. Thus, conditions affecting CBG production, such as thyroid disease or liver cirrhosis indirectly alter free cortisol levels [71]. Additionally, CBG levels seem to fall in response to acute stress, possibly freeing additional amounts of cortisol [72]. The free hormone concept, however, has recently been challenged [73, 74]. In some circumstances, such as local inflammation, it has been shown that CBG may selectively deliver cortisol to a target site and therefore may also exert an active role. Therefore, the precise role of CBG within chronic stress remains somewhat unclear; however, it is certain that CBG alterations are very important to HPA functioning and CBG should thus be routinely assessed in HPA research.

4.2.3. Compensation

At any point of the outlined regulatory excitatory or inhibitory endocrine pathways, compensatory mechanisms can operate in a self-adjusting way to dampen overactive signaling. Accordingly, with regard to receptors (CRF receptor, melanocortin receptor, GR, MR) or plasma/cytosolic binding proteins (CRF-binding protein, CBG) up- and downregulations in number or sensitivity are frequently described [75, 76].

4.3. Endophenotypes

In the following, we introduce the neuropattern approach focusing on interfaces related to HPAA hyperactivity. First, we differentiate between central nervous system components, i.e. paraventricular CRF hypersecretion and peripheral alterations such as increased adrenal glucocorticoid output. On the central level, we then further distinguish between state and trait components of CRF hypersecretion: the first refers to basal HPA upregulation, termed CRF hyperactivity (see 4.3.1.), while the latter comprises enhanced reactions to stress, termed CRF hyperreactivity (see 4.3.2.).

4.3.1. CRF Hyperactivity

We conceptualize CRF hyperactivity as a state of increased CRF secretion from parvocellular CRF neurons originating in the PVN and leading down to the median eminence. Reaching the pituitary portal system, CRF is carried to the anterior pituitary lobe, where it elicits POMC processing and ACTH generation in corticotropes through binding at CRF receptors. CRF hyperactivity denotes a state of basal as well as stress-related hypothalamic and, in many cases, consequent pituitary overdrive, coinciding with a spectrum of CRF-mediated psychological and physiological consequences.

As CRF effects underlie classical conditioning [77], it can be assumed that mere cognitions may independently elicit the whole range of CRF-mediated endocrine and autonomous reactions. Also, anticipatory worrying about one's own position in a given social, spatial, and temporal context may effectively activate the hippocampus and eventually hypothalamic CRF neurons [78, 79]. Phenotypically, these experiences present as recurring anticipatory ruminations and worries.

At the pituitary level, the acute bodily response to CRF overexpression would be CRF receptor downregulation at corticotropes, which partly dampens the CRF signal [80]. In the long-run, pituitary CRF receptor downregulation is considered adaptive to chronic paraventricular CRF hypersecretion. Thus, one can expect that ACTH release is still but only moderately enhanced [81, 82]. In humans, CRF hyperactivity cannot be measured in a direct manner; however, an indirect approach is to estimate ACTH output to a bolus i.v. injection of CRF [83]. When followed by a blunted ACTH response, receptor downregulation may be assumed. Another way to target such alterations is to measure ACTH secretion in consequence to a psychosocial stress challenge. However, it cannot be excluded that severely stressed people such as victims of violence may process a mild laboratory stressor in an entirely different way, i.e. laboratory stress may not elicit a measurable stress response given its blandness compared to real life stressors. Thus, results obtained with laboratory stress should be interpreted in a deliberate way. A third way, although not too practicable in most cases, is to assess liquor probes. However, while being a direct measure of CRF, they carry the disadvantage of being a mixture of what is produced in the circumventricular brain structures without offering site specificity. A fourth measure in human research, and even less useful, is to assess CRF concentrations and CRF mRNA in postmortem tissue.

Typical CRF-mediated symptoms include loss of appetite, inhibition of reproductive functioning, increased vigilance, sleep disorders, anxiety and depression [7]. Generally, peripheral glucocorticoid status should be assessed and taken into account, as glucocorticoids often act synergistically, but at different levels.

4.3.1.1. Loss of Appetite

Paraventricular CRF plays a part within the intricate neuronal network regulating appetite, though its role has not yet been entirely elucidated. Cardinal hypothalamic loci involved in feeding and satiety signaling (i.e. the arcuate nucleus, dorsomedial hypothalamus, ventromedial hypothalamus) send efferents to the PVN and partly to its parvocellular subdivision; however, it appears that the PVN itself is only of second-order importance and rather mediates incoming signals emitted from the formerly named nuclei. In rats, i.c.v. injection of CRF has an anorexigenic effect and the site of action has been traced to mainly be the PVN. CRF locally injected into the PVN inhibits fasting-induced as well as NPY-induced feeding. Local administration of α-helical CRF, a CRF antagonist, recompensates the anorexigenic effect of CRF, when administered directly into the PVN, but not when given into the ventromedial hypothalamus, indicating the involvement of local PVN CRF receptors. Furthermore, injections of either orexigenic or anorexigenic substances elicit increased c-FOS activation, an indicator of early gene activation, in PVN neurons. In animal models, PVN lesioning leads to hyperphagia and body weight gain. It is assumed, however, that these effects are due to local CRF secretion within the hypothalamus (for review, see [84]). In chronic fasting, however, paraventricular CRF signaling is highly enhanced [85].

4.3.1.2. Inhibition of Reproductive Functions

CRF also inhibits the hypothalamic-pituitary-gonadal axis at a central level, a phenomenon known in women as hypothalamic amenorrhea. Gonadotropin-releasing hormone (GnRH) neurons located throughout the hypothalamic preoptic region project to the median eminence, where GnRH is released into the hypophyseal portal circulation. In female rats, i.c.v. injections of CRF dampen GnRH levels in the portal bloodstream [86] and dose-dependently decrease luteinizing hormone (LH) secretion in ovariectomized rats [87]. In freely cycling female rats, after restraint stress (5 h), the proestrus LH surge as well as ovulation is inhibited [88].

As exercise activates the HPAA akin to stress, similar mechanisms have been assumed for highly trained female athletes [89] and for patients with anorexia nervosa [90], both of whom frequently suffer from amenorrhea. Chronic CRF secretion may thus predispose to infertility and alterations in the female cycle.

4.3.1.3. Anxiety

Paraventricular CRF neurons are positively interconnected with noradrenergic fibers originating in the LC (see 4.2. and chapters 3, 7), which are assumed to play an important role in attention processes and vigilance [38, 43, 91]. In response to chronic CRF hypersecretion, these processes may be getting overstretched, shifting from a 'good' state of attentiveness to a state of overexcitation and stimulus overprocessing.

Corroborating evidence stems from animal experiments, in which administration of CRF into the CNS produces anxiety-like effects in a variety of measures [81]. Similarly, either in animals that were treated with CRF antagonists or that stem from a CRF receptor 1 knockout strain, anxyiolytic behavioral effects are evident. It is speculated, however, that these effects are secondarily mediated via stimulation of noradrenergic brain networks (see chapter 6).

4.3.1.4. Irritable Stomach and Irritable Bowel Syndrome

Central CRF secretion inhibits gastric emptying, while stimulating colonic motility through alterations in the parasympathetic nervous system (i.e. n. vagus and sacral efferences). While CRF projections from the PVN are involved in both processes, the first additionally engages the dorsal vagal complex and the latter the LC. CRF activation appears to mediate stress-induced fecation and gastrointestinal symptoms characteristic for the irritable bowel syndrome [32].

4.3.1.5. Melancholic Depression

In multiple studies, CRF hyperactivity has been assessed in patients with major depression. Stressful events seem to promote the onset of depressive episodes and appear to aggravate depressive symptoms. Increased levels of CRF have been found in postmortem brain tissue of severely depressed suicide victims as well as in cerebrospinal fluid (CSF) samples, while CRF receptor-binding sites were decreased in the prefrontal cortices of suicide victims. On the other hand, either electroconvulsive therapy or the use of antidepressants normalizes both depressive symptoms and CRF levels in the CSF. Depressive patients show blunted ACTH responses in reaction to exogenous CRF (i.v.), indicative of a compensatory downregulation due to chronic endogenous CRF overstimulation [81, 92]. With amelioration of depressive symptoms, ACTH levels to CRF stimulation also normalize [93], suggesting a functional relationship between both phenomena.

Generally, CRF hyperreactivity is probably only prevalent in a clinical subgroup of patients with depression. It appears that it is mostly persons who insufficiently suppress cortisol in response to dexamethasone stimulation who may fall into this group

[94]. Interestingly, there are indications that this subgroup is particularly at risk of committing suicide [95]. It is suggested that typical CRF-mediated symptoms are particularly evident in one subtype called melancholic depression: patients with the melancholic subtype of depression present with overexcitation, loss of libido, loss of appetite, infertility and sleeping disorders [7]. Still, the biopsychological differentiation of clinical subgroups in depression deserves further attention and should be further elucidated in the future.

4.3.2. CRF Hyperreactivity

CRF hyperreactivity refers to a state characterized by increased HPA reactivity to psychological stress, while basal HPA activity remains within the normal range. We expect that the most prominent brain structure conveying this disparity is the hippocampus. Binding of glucocorticoids in the hippocampus plays a predominant role in suppressing CRF secretion in the PVN, as could be shown in animal experiments using different experimental paradigms, such as hippocampal lesioning, electrical stimulation, GR blockade and corticosterone implants [96]. Dysfunctions in the hippocampus may therefore impair inhibitory glucocorticoid feedback actions resulting in a stress-sensitive phenotype. Still, negative feedback regulation of the HPAA is stressor-specific (see above). Hence, hippocampally mediated feedback operates in more 'psychological' stress such as, in animal experiments, novelty or restraint stress as opposed to more 'physiological' stress such as hypoxia [97]. In humans, hippocampal activation of CRF release may particularly occur when the organism is confronted with stressors characterized as highly ambiguous, novel, unpredictable and uncontrollable [98, 99]. A meta-analysis of more than 200 studies employing different laboratory stress paradigms in humans concluded that those stress inductions were most efficient in eliciting cortisol responses, which evoked a high amount of uncontrollability paired with social evaluative threat [100].

The hippocampus also seems to be involved in mediating the cortisol response to awakening: hippocampectomy in humans abolishes the distinct rise in cortisol within the first 30 min after awakening [101]. Its precise role in regulating circadian cortisol secretion, however, remains to be elucidated. Impaired hippocampal control of HPA regulation due to a lack of hippocampal GR expression has been found as a consequence of early postnatal adversity (see below). Particularly, the meanwhile famous rodent model studied by Michael Meaney's group in Montreal lends strong evidence to this hypothesis [21, 27, 28]. In this model, changes in hippocampal GR expression have been traced back to alterations in the epigenome (see above). Of note, they are entirely reversible through cross-fostering, indicating a merely behaviorally mediated effect by the degree of postnatal maternal care. Hence, in the early phases of brain maturation, such processes may play a pivotal role for the developing organism, which may then lay the cornerstone for future developmental trajectories.

Concerning human research, beginning with the seminal studies of Barker et al. [102, 103], a panoply of studies has examined prenatal adversities, such as effects of malnutrition, maternal infection or prenatal stress, on the long-term development of HPAA functioning. Early adverse events are now considered a major source of vulnerability for the development of stress-related psychopathologies and medical conditions such as depression, diabetes mellitus type 2, cardiovascular disease, insulin resistance and obesity [103–107]. Alterations in brain functioning and HPAA regulation are considered the cardinal factors predisposing to these unfavorable bodily conditions [20]. However, the majority of studies focus on uterine growth restriction, assessing birth weight, gestational length and/or gestational age. Prenatal psychosocial stress, per se, has received less scientific attention. Still, physiological stress (i.e. infections, hypoxia, malnutrition) and psychosocial stress may basically be comparable [22]. Psychosocial stress, maternal infection, malnutrition or some other placental disorders may all exert their adverse effects through fetal overexposure of stress hormones such as glucocorticoids/catecholamines or through cutting the fetus off from sufficient oxygen and nutrient supply due to placental vasoconstriction. Furthermore, postnatal adversities early in childhood such as abuse, violence or separation from a parent may induce comparable HPAA alterations. However, what remains a matter of debate is the time frame within early development, in which stress evokes long-lasting alterations, which seem to be qualitatively different from the timing in pregnancy.

Prenatal stress may be related to increased HPA activity to stress, insulin resistance and other mental health impairments. In a study of 106 male twins, Wust et al. [12] found that birth weight was inversely related to the salivary cortisol reaction to psychosocial stress (TSST). This result is in line with findings from other laboratories that used birth weight as a proxy for adverse uterine processes putatively programming HPA hyperactivity. Entringer [108] found that prenatal stress was significantly associated with insulin resistance in the oral glucose tolerance test, remarkably even in a sample of healthy students. Of note, no group differences in birth weight were reported; hence, prenatal stress may not necessarily translate into overt uterine growth restriction. Insulin resistance is a risk factor for developing diabetes mellitus type 2 later in life [109]. Interestingly, patients with diabetes mellitus type 2 display dysfunctions in declarative memory, a marker for hippocampus functioning influenced by glucocorticoids [110]. In another study, HbA1c levels, an indicator for blood glucose levels within the last 3 months, were significantly associated with hippocampal volume loss, accounting for 33% of the variance. Causality between both phenomenons, however, remains unclear.

First results from an extended longitudinal study in Great Britain indicate that prenatal stress, particularly problems with the partner during pregnancy, are related to higher anxiety levels, language delay and an increased risk for the development of attention deficit and hyperactivity disorder (ADHD) in the child. To what concerns early postnatal adversities and HPA alterations in humans, information is still lacking [111].

In terms of cortisol secretion, we are postulating two main scenarios in consequence of early adversities:

(1) We expect that in some individuals, prenatal psychological stress exposure such as separation/divorce from the husband/partner during pregnancy or loss of a significant other during pregnancy may lead to persisting disruptions in HPA functioning similar to alterations described for low birth weight, which is well examined in the literature. We think that in the adult, alterations due to prenatal stress present as CRF hyperreactivity and are mainly due to persisting alterations in regulatory brain structures such as the hippocampus. We therefore assume that basal cortisol may remain relatively unaffected, while cortisol responses to stress as well as to awakening are considerably elevated. Cortisol suppression to dexamethasone, as shown in the low-dose dexamethasone suppression test, is expected to be in the normal-to-low range.

(2) We assume a second endophenotype in consequence of early life stress (probably in the first trimester of pregnancy), which affects only a small group (approximately 2–3%) of subjects. Here, cortisol hypersecretion due to CRF hyperreactivity is compensated by the development of an intensified negative feedback signal at the pituitary level. Thus, only under stress and during the diurnal cortisol peak in the morning is HPAA hyperreactivity evident, while basal cortisol levels otherwise remain in the normal-to-low range. After dexamethasone, however, a supersuppression of cortisol levels will be observed [Kajantie, Phillips, Hellhammer, unpubl.]. As a consequence, hypercortisolemic disorders, e.g. as in group 1, should not occur, but we expect that somatic and mental fatigue may be expressed, probably mediated by cytokines. When reanalyzing our in-house patient sample of subjects suffering from mental and physical fatigue (n = 47), this pattern occurred in 30% of the subjects. Interestingly, this group particularly suffers from muscle fatigue as opposed to mental fatigue [Hellhammer, unpubl.]. CRF hyperreactivity with increased feedback sensitivity to 0.25 mg overnight dexamethasone may thus describe a distinct subgroup of patients primarily affected by fatigue and pain syndromes.

Case Report

Our patient (22 years of age, weight 60 kg, height 1.74 m) presented with severe muscle fatigue, persisting for 8 years. The ailments started after an episode of bullying by classmates during puberty, and never entirely faded since, though phases of amelioration alternated with phases of relapse. Fatigue severity worsened in the morning, during infectious disease, after psychological stress and after glucocorticoid intake (prednisolone). In summary, this description suggests an association of symptom severity with glucocorticoid levels, with symptom deterioration related to phases of high glucocorticoid secretion.

For 8 years, the patient received numerous diagnostic and therapeutic treatments (e.g. muscle biopsies, antidepressants, psychotherapy) without any real success. Finally, he was told to accept the diagnosis of a 'somatoform disorder', and his insurance company refused to cover any other treatment costs.

The patient then underwent the neuropattern diagnostics and qualified for 'CRF hyperreactivity': within the course of the first trimester of pregnancy, his mother, while suffering from severe pregnancy-related vomiting and vertigo, had lost 7 kg. When born, the patient had a relatively low birth weight of 3,040 g. In support of this, the patient showed an extremely high awakening response (58 nmol/l), but a supersuppression to dexamethasone.

In order to further examine HPAA functioning in this patient, we assessed seven basal diurnal cortisol profiles and three diurnal profiles after premedication with dexamethasone. Compared to 20 healthy men of the same age, his cortisol levels in response to awakening were always highly elevated, while the basal diurnal cortisol secretion was conserved. Cortisol levels after dexamethasone were fully suppressed, indicating increased sensitivity to glucocorticoid negative feedback actions at the level of the pituitary. Also, catecholamine levels were conspicuously elevated in response to the TSST. Examination of his endocrine reaction to the TSST revealed an interesting picture: while serum cortisol levels remained in the normal range (after starting at a very low basal value), serum ACTH and free cortisol levels rose exorbitantly high. When measuring his CBG levels, a very low value was assessed (29.7 vs. 39.7 ± 6.3 μg/ml), explaining the obvious disparity between protein-bound and free cortisol levels. Further analyses revealed a very rare mutation within the SERPINA6 gene (Lyon mutation), leading to dysfunctional CBG protein with low cortisol affinity.*

Our diagnostics thus offered the following explanation for his health problems: First, one can assume that prenatal stress resulted (perhaps via methylation of the hippocampal GR gene) in a disinhibition of the PVN to stress. Thus, the patient showed an enhanced HPAA response to both awakening and laboratory stress. The assumption of a CRF hyperreactivity was supported by concomitant response of catecholamines to stress. In addition, the high cortisol responses to stress could not be buffered by CBG, due to the CBG gene mutation. Thus, any daily stressor could result in high glucocorticoid effects on target tissues, provoking his symptomatology.

* Buss C, Schuetter U, Hesse J, Moser D, Phillips DI, Hellhammer D, Meyer J: Haploinsufficiency of the SERPINA6 gene is associated with severe muscle fatigue: a de novo mutation in corticosteroid-binding globulin deficiency. J Neural Transm 2007;114:563–569.

Our case illustrates the complexity and heterogeneity of stress-related disorders and the necessity of personalized diagnostics and treatment (see chapter 2). Since his prenatally programmed endocrine pattern is rare, and Lyon mutations are moreover extremely rare, even large deductive research studies would be unable to generate a subgroup of such patients. Finally, we feel that many 'somatoform disorders' have a chance to be uncovered in the individual, once the currently available knowledge can be translated to clinical practice.

4.3.3. Cortisol Hyperactivity

We define 'cortisol hyperactivity' as an enhanced efficacy of cortisol on target tissues in consequence of either cortisol overexposure or increased effects of cortisol on its receptors. While the former may be due to an increased adrenal capacity and/or an increased adrenal sensitivity to ACTH, the latter comprises alterations in cortisol receptors.

4.3.3.1. Increased Adrenal Capacity

As known from Selye's early work, chronic stress can induce hypertrophy (increased cell size) and subsequently hyperplasia (increased cell number) of adrenal tissue with consequently increased cortisol secretion to a stimulus [3, 69, 112]. Also, adrenal tumor growth or increased sympathetic stimulation conveyed through the adrenal medulla may cause an increase in the secretion or liberation of cortisol [113]. Adrenal capacity is defined as the maximal cortisol output to stimulation with a pharmacological amount of ACTH [83]. In order to experimentally quantify adrenal capacity, subjects are given a bolus injection of ACTH (250 μg i.v.) and the subsequent cortisol release from the adrenals is assessed.

A study on melancholic depression recently showed that hypercortisolism can coincide with normal CRF and ACTH levels in the CSF [114]. Also, increased CSF norepinephrine levels were observed in this study. As it is known that the splanchnic nerve of the sympathetic nervous system innervates the adrenal medulla, sympathetic arousal can remarkably potentiate ACTH-elicited cortisol secretion under stress conditions, and it seems possible that chronic ergotropic stress may increase adrenal capacity [115, 116].

Another putative source of adrenal hyperactivity consists of a prenatally determined alteration in cortisol metabolism, a hypothesis which is still currently under investigation [Seckl, pers. commun.].

Adrenal capacity appears to share common features with the cortisol rise after awakening, as has been shown in a study on healthy young volunteers: Schmidt-Reinwald et al. [117] reported a significant correlation ($r = 0.63$) between the cortisol increase to awakening and adrenal capacity, while no such associations were found with regard to responses to psychosocial stress or stimulation with exogenous CRF.

4.3.3.2. Adrenal Sensitivity

As opposed to adrenal capacity, adrenal sensitivity signifies the cortisol response to a minimal and rather physiological stimulation with ACTH, giving the opportunity to study more subtle differences in HPA regulation, as is desired in investigating stress-related disorders such as fibromyalgia or chronic fatigue syndrome [118, 119], but which may also be of interest in the analysis of subtle hypercortisolemic dysregulations. Adrenal sensitivity can be estimated as the cortisol response to a minor dose of exogenous ACTH (1 μg i.v.).

4.3.3.3. Downregulation of Glucocorticoid Receptors on Lymphocytes

A potential consequence of cortisol hypersecretion may be the downregulation of its target glucocorticoid receptors. The GR status on lymphocytes has been measured under various conditions associated with increased cortisol secretion, such as strenuous exercise [120] and dexamethasone administration [121]. Whether such alterations may serve as a model for CNS processes remains elusive. Still, GR regulation also displays tissue specificity, so this model should not be used without careful analysis of one's underlying assumptions [122, 123].

4.3.3.4. Sequelae of Cortisol Hypersecretion

Chronic HPA activity may lead to a host of adverse physiological consequences altering the biological systems responsible for reproduction, growth and development, feeding, mood, and cardiovascular, thyroid and immune system functioning (for review, see [5, 6]). It is, however, difficult to disentangle effects due to CRF hyperactivity and effects due to cortisol hypersecretion. To take gonadal functioning as an example, CRF inhibits hypothalamic centers liberating gonadotropin-releasing hormone, while glucocorticoids inhibit pituitary gonadotropes, the gonads themselves as well as sex hormone target tissues.

4.3.3.5. Metabolism

Accumulating evidence in animals and humans indicates that abdominal obesity as well as other adverse metabolic alterations such as insulin resistance, hyperinsulinemia and impaired glucose tolerance may result from HPA hyperactivity after chronic exposure to stress. In animals, adrenal hyperplasia and increased cortisol secretion to ACTH was found in obese subjects. Truncal fat accumulation is also a cardinal sign of Cushing syndrome or prolonged high-dose glucocorticoid treatment.

In the liver, cortisol increases gluconeogenesis, while in the presence of insulin, accumulation of fat in the abdomen is triggered. Cortisol increases preadipocyte differentiation and inhibits glucose uptake in peripheral tissue, while enhancing the conversion of free fatty acids to central fat depots. Also, higher levels of GR are found in abdominal fat compared to subcutaneous fat tissue, rendering it selectively more susceptible to glucocorticoid effects. Furthermore, altered enzyme status indicates chronic cortisol excess: activity of 11β-HSD1, responsible for reactivating cortisol from its biologically passive form cortisone as well as enhancing activities in enzymes occupied with cortisol degradation, such as 5-α-reductase, have been reported in obese subjects. Furthermore, insulin metabolism is altered by a variety of mechanisms, such as affecting glucose transporter function in insulin-sensitive tissues [124]. Other than that, stressful life conditions such as low socioeconomic status, high perceived stress, or negative health behaviors elicited by stress (smoking, drinking, drug abuse) are significantly more frequent in individuals with abdominal obesity. Still, HPA hyperactivity is not a unique sign of obesity. Conflicting findings indicate that only a subgroup of obese patients is affected by HPA alterations (for review, see [125, 126]).

4.3.3.6. Depression

HPA dysregulations in major depression may also be primarily regarded from the perspective of peripheral glucocorticoid output rather than central CRF hypersecretion, though both mechanisms may go hand in hand. Antiglucocorticoid treatment efficiently reduces depressive symptomatology, as has been shown for DHEA, steroid synthesis inhibitors and glucocorticoid antagonists [127]. In a subtype of depression called psychotic major depression, high-dose treatment with the progesterone antagonist mifepristone (RU 486) has shown to be useful. While originally mifepristone was developed as an early abortifacient, it was found that at higher doses, it contains strong antiglucocorticoid properties, acting at the glucocorticoid receptors. It is hypothesized that RU 486 mainly provokes a rapid increase in GR number, thus improving negative feedback actions. Another potential mechanism may be the restoration of MR numbers affecting basal HPA functioning [127–129].

41 Chrousos GP: Regulation and dysregulation of the hypothalamic-pituitary-adrenal axis: the corticotropin-releasing hormone perspective. Endocrinol Metab Clin N Am 1992;21:833–858.
42 Dunn AJ, Swiergiel AH, Palamarchouk V: Brain circuits involved in corticotropin-releasing factor-norepinephrine interactions during stress. Ann NY Acad Sci 2004;1018:25–34.
43 Aston-Jones G, Rajkowski J, Kubiak P, Valentino RJ, Shipley MT: Role of the locus coeruleus in emotional activation. Prog Brain Res 1996;107:379–402.
44 Dallman MF: Fast glucocorticoid feedback favors 'the munchies'. Trends Endocrinol Metab 2003;14: 394–396.
45 Dallman MF: Glucocorticoid negative feedback; in Fink G (ed): Encyclopedia of Stress. San Diego, Academic Press, 2000, pp 224–228.
46 Dallman MF: Fast glucocorticoid actions on brain: back to the future. Front Neuroendocrinol 2005;26: 103–108.
47 Dallman MF, Pecoraro NC, la Fleur SE: Chronic stress and comfort foods: self-medication and abdominal obesity. Brain Behav Immun 2005;19:275–280.
48 Di S, Malcher-Lopes R, Halmos KC, Tasker JG: Nongenomic glucocorticoid inhibition via endocannabinoid release in the hypothalamus: a fast feedback mechanism. J Neurosci 2003;23:4850–4857.
49 Tasker JG, Di S, Malcher-Lopes R: Rapid central corticosteroid effects: Evidence for membrane glucocorticoid receptor in the brain. Integr Comp Biol 2005;45:665–671.
50 Dallman MF, Pecoraro NC, La Fleur SE, Warne JP, Ginsberg AB, Akana SF, Laugero KC, Houshyar H, Strack AM, Bhatnagar S, Bell ME: Glucocorticoids, chronic stress and obesity; in Kalsbeek A, Fliers E (eds): Hypothalamic Integration of Energy Metabolism. Amsterdam, Elsevier, 2005, pp 75–106.
51 McEwen BS: Protection and damage from acute and chronic stress: allostasis and allostatic overload and relevance to the pathophysiology of psychiatric disorders. Ann NY Acad Sci 2004;1032:1–7.
52 Korte SM, Koolhaas JM, Wingfield JC, McEwen BS: The Darwinian concept of stress: benefits of allostasis and costs of allostatic load and the trade-offs in health and disease. Neurosci Biobehav Rev 2005; 29:3–38.
53 Schommer NC: Das Ausmaß endokriner und kardiovaskulärer Reaktionen infolge wiederholter psychosozialer Belastung: ein Prädiktor für zukünftige gesundheitliche Beeinträchtigung? Diss, Göttingen, Cuvillier Verlag, 2002.
54 Dallman MF, Akana SF, Cascio CS, Darlington DN, Jacobson L, Levin N: Regulation of ACTH secretion: variations on a theme of B. Recent Prog Horm Res 1987;43:113–173.
55 Dallman MF, Pecoraro N, Akana SF, La Fleur SE, Gomez F, Houshyar H, Bell ME, Bhatnagar S, Laugero KD, Manalo S: Chronic stress and obesity: a new view of 'comfort food'. Proc Natl Acad Sci USA 2003;100:11696–11701.
56 Dallman MF, Viau VG, Bhatnagar S, Gomez F, Laugero K, Bell ME: Corticotropin-releasing factor, corticosteroids, stress and sugar: energy balance, the brain, and behavior; in Pfaff DW, Arnold AP, Etgen AM, Fahrbach SE, Rubin RT (eds): Hormones, Brain and Behavior. San Diego, Academic Press, 2002, pp 571–632.
57 Schulkin J, Gold PW, McEwen BS: Induction of corticotropin-releasing hormone gene expression by glucocorticoids: implication for understanding the states of fear and anxiety and allostatic load. Psychoneuroendocrinology 1998;23:219–243.
58 Schulkin J, McEwen BS, Gold PW: Allostasis, amygdala, and anticipatory angst. Neurosci Biobehav Rev 1994;18:385–396.
59 Merali Z, McIntosh J, Kent P, Michaud D, Anisman H: Aversive and appetitive events evoke the release of corticotropin-releasing hormone and bombesin-like peptides at the central nucleus of the amygdala. J Neurosci 1998;18:4758–4766.
60 Merlo Pich E, Lorang M, Yeganeh M, Rodriguez de Fonseca F, Raber J, Koob GF, Weiss F: Increase of extracellular corticotropin-releasing factor-like immunoreactivity levels in the amygdala of awake rats during restraint stress and ethanol withdrawal as measured by microdialysis. J Neurosci 1995;15: 5439–5447.
61 Shalev U, Morales M, Hope B, Yap J, Shaham Y: Time-dependent changes in extinction behavior and stress-induced reinstatement of drug seeking following withdrawal from heroin in rats. Psychopharmacology (Berl) 2001;156:98–107.
62 Wilensky AE, Schafe GE, Kristensen MP, LeDoux JE. Rethinking the fear circuit: the central nucleus of the amygdala is required for the acquisition, consolidation, and expression of Pavlovian fear conditioning. J Neurosci 2006;26:12387–12396.
63 Davis M, Whalen PJ: The amygdala: vigilance and emotion. Mol Psychiatry 2001;6:13–34.
64 Heinrichs SC, Pich EM, Miczek KA, Britton KT, Koob GF: Corticotropin-releasing factor antagonist reduces emotionality in socially defeated rats via direct neurotropic action. Brain Res 1992;581: 190–197.
65 Swiergiel AH, Takahashi LK, Kalin NH: Attenuation of stress-induced behavior by antagonism of corticotropin-releasing factor receptors in the central amygdala in the rat. Brain Res 1993;623:229–234.

66 Antoni FA: Vasopressinergic control of pituitary adrenocorticotropin secretion comes of age. Front Neuroendocrinol 1993;14:76–122.
67 Gillies GE, Linton EA, Lowry PJ: Corticotropin releasing activity of the new CRF is potentiated several times by vasopressin. Nature 1982;299:355–357.
68 Lim MC, Shipston MJ, Antoni FA: Posttranslational modulation of glucocorticoid feedback inhibition at the pituitary level. Endocrinology 2002;143:3796–3801.
69 Ulrich-Lai YM, Figueiredo HF, Ostrander MM, Choi DC, Engeland WC, Herman JP: Chronic stress induces adrenal hyperplasia and hypertrophy in a subregion-specific manner. Am J Physiol 2006;291:E965–E973.
70 Mendel CM: The free hormone hypothesis; distinction from the free hormone transport hypothesis. J Androl 1992;13:107–116.
71 Hatz HJ: Glucocorticoide. Stuttgart, Wissenschaftliche Verlagsgesellschaft, 2005.
72 Fleshner M, Deak T, Spencer RL, Laudenslager ML, Watkins LR, Maier SF: A long-term increase in basal levels of corticosterone and a decrease in corticosteroid-binding globulin after acute stressor exposure. Endocrinology 1995;136:5336–5342.
73 Breuner CW, Orchinik M: Plasma binding proteins as mediators of corticosteroid action in vertebrates. J Endocrinol 2002;175:99–112.
74 Petersen HH, Andreassen TK, Breiderhoff T, Brasen JH, Schulz H, Gross V, Grone HJ, Nykjaer A, Willnow TE: Hyporesponsiveness to glucocorticoids in mice genetically deficient for the corticosteroid binding globulin. Mol Cell Biol 2006;26:7236–7245.
75 Hellhammer DH, Wade S: Endocrine correlates of stress vulnerability. Psychother Psychosom 1993;60:8–17.
76 Fink G: Feedback systems; in: Encyclopedia of Stress. Academic Press, 2000, pp 124–158.
77 Kreutz M, Hellhammer D, Murison R, Vetter H, Krause U, Lehnert H: Pavlovian conditioning of corticotropin-releasing factor-induced increase of blood pressure and corticosterone secretion in the rat. Acta Physiol Scand 1992;145:59–63.
78 Hellhammer DH: Gehirn und Verhalten: Eine anwendungsorientierte Einführung in die Psychobiologie. Münster, Aschendorff, 1983.
79 Mason JW: A review of psychoendocrine research on the pituitary-adrenal cortical system. Psychosom Medicine 1968;30:576–607.
80 Hauger RL, Millan MA, Lorang M, Harwood JP, Aguilera G: Corticotropin-releasing factor receptors and pituitary adrenal responses during immobilization stress. Endocrinology 1988;123:396–405.
81 Arborelius L, Owens MJ, Plotsky PM, Nemeroff CB: The role of corticotropin-releasing factor in depression and anxiety disorders. J Endocrinol 1999;160:1–12.
82 O'Connor KA, Ginsberg AB, Maksimova E, Wieseler Frank JL, Johnson JD, Spencer RL, Campeau S, Watkins LR, Maier SF: Stress-induced sensitization of the hypothalamic-pituitary adrenal axis is associated with alterations of hypothalamic and pituitary gene expression. Neuroendocrinology 2004;80:252–263.
83 Heim C, Ehlert U: Pharmakologische Provokationstests zur Einschätzung der neuroendokrinen Funktionen; in Kirschbaum C, Hellhammer D (eds): Enzyklopädie der Psychologie, Bd. 3: Psychoendokrinologie und Psychoimmunologie. Göttingen, Hogrefe, 1999, pp 307–346.
84 Kalra SP, Dube MG, Pu S, Xu B, Horvath TL, Kalra PS: Interacting appetite-regulating pathways in the hypothalamic regulation of body weight. Endocr Rev 1999;20:68–100.
85 Dallman MF, Akana SF, Bhatnagar S, Bell ME, Choi S, Chu A, Horsley C, Levin N, Meijer O, Soriano LR, Strack AM, Viau V: Starvation: early signals, sensors, and sequelae. Endocrinology 1999;140:4015–4023.
86 Petraglia F, Florio P, Nappi C, Genazzani AR: Peptide signaling in human placenta and membranes: autocrine, paracrine and endocrine mechanism. Endocr Rev 1996;17:156–186.
87 Rivier C, Vale W: Influence of corticotropin-releasing factor on reproductive functions in the rat. Endocrinology 1984;114:914–921.
88 Roozendaal MM, Swarts HJ, Wiegant VM, Mattheij JA: Effect of restraint stress on the preovulatory luteinizing hormone profile and ovulation in the rat. Eur J Endocrinol 1995;133:347–353.
89 Mastorakos G, Pavlatou M, Diamanti-Kandarakis E, Chrousos GP: Exercise and the stress system. Hormones (Athens) 2005;4:73–89.
90 Munoz MT, Argente J: Anorexia nervosa in female adolescents: endocrine and bone mineral density disturbances. Eur J Endocrinol 2002;147:275–286.
91 Aston-Jones G, Bloom FE: Nonrepinephrine-containing locus coeruleus neurons in behaving rats exhibit pronounced responses to non-noxious environmental stimuli. J Neurosci 1981;1:887–900.
92 Holsboer F, Muller OA, Doerr HG, Sippell WG, Stalla GK, Gerken A, Steiger A, Boll E, Benkert O: ACTH and multisteroid responses to corticotropin-releasing factor in depressive illness: relationship to multisteroid responses after ACTH stimulation and dexamethasone suppression. Psychoneuroendocrinology 1984;9:147–160.

93 Amsterdam JD, Maislin G, Winokur A, Berwish N, Kling M, Gold P: The oCRH stimulation test before and after clinical recovery from depression. J Affect Disord 1988;14:213–222.
94 Roy A, Pickar D, Paul S, Doran A, Chrousos GP, Gold PW: CSF corticotropin-releasing hormone in depressed patients and normal control subjects. Am J Psychiatry 1987;144:641–645.
95 Coryell W, Schlesser M: The dexamethasone suppression test and suicide prediction. Am J Psychiatry 2001;158:748–753.
96 Jacobson L, Sapolsky R: The role of the hippocampus in feedback regulation of the hypothalamic-pituitary-adrenocortical axis. Endocr Rev 1991; 12:118–134.
97 Ziegler DR, Herman JP: Neurocircuitry of stress integration: anatomical pathways regulating the hypothalamo-pituitary-adrenocortical axis of the rat. Integ and Comp Biol 2002;42:541–551.
98 Mason JW: A review of psychoendocrine research on the pituitary-adrenal cortical system. Psychosom Med 1968;30(suppl):576–607.
99 Huppmann G, Hellhammer D: Aspects of anxiety-fear differentiation. Z Klin Psychol Psychother 1978;26:115–127.
100 Dickerson SS, Kemeny ME: Acute stressors and cortisol responses: a theoretical integration and synthesis of laboratory research. Psychol Bull 2004;130:355–391.
101 Buchanan TW, Kern S, Allen JS, Tranel D, Kirschbaum C: Circadian regulation of cortisol after hippocampal damage in humans. Biol Psychiatry 2004;56:651–656.
102 Barker DJ: Intrauterine programming of adult disease. Mol Med Today 1995;1:418–423.
103 Barker DJ: Maternal and fetal origins of coronary heart disease. J R Coll Physns Lond 1994;28:544–551.
104 Eriksson JG, Forsen T, Tuomilehto J, Osmond C, Barker DJ: Early growth and coronary heart disease in later life: longitudinal study. BMJ 2001;322: 949–953.
105 Barker DJ: Fetal programming of coronary heart disease. Trends Endocrinol Metab 2002;13:364–368.
106 Phillips DI, Barker DJ, Fall CH, Seckl JR, Whorwood CB, Wood PJ, Walker BR: Elevated plasma cortisol concentrations: a link between low birth weight and the insulin resistance syndrome? J Clin Endocrinol Metab 1998;83:757–760.
107 Phillips DI, Walker BR, Reynolds RM, Flanagan DE, Wood PJ, Osmond C, Barker DJ, Whorwood CB: Low birth weight predicts elevated plasma cortisol concentrations in adults from 3 populations. Hypertension 2000;35:1301–1306.
108 Entringer S: Exposure to Prenatal Stress: Implications for Long-term Disease Susceptibility. Göttingen, Cuvillier, 2007.
109 Twigg SM, Kamp MC, Davis TM, Neylon EK, Flack JR: Prediabetes: a position statement from the Australian Diabetes Society and Australian Diabetes Educators Association. Med J Aust 2007; 186:461–465.
110 Bruehl H, Rueger M, Dziobek I, Sweat V, Tirsi A, Javier E, Arentoft A, Wolf OT, Convit A: Hypothalamic-pituitary-adrenal axis dysregulation and memory impairments in type 2 diabetes. J Clin Endocrinol Metab 2007;92:2439–2445.
111 Sanchez MM, Ladd CO, Plotsky PM: Early adverse experience as a developmental risk factor for later psychopathology: evidence from rodent and primate models. Dev Psychopathol 2001;13:419–449.
112 Dallman MF: Control of adrenocortical growth in vivo. Endocr Res 1984;10:213–242.
113 Ehrhart-Bornstein M, Hinson JP, Bornstein SR, Scherbaum WA, Vinson GP: Intraadrenal interactions in the regulation of adrenocortical steroidogenesis. Endocr Rev 1998;19:101–143.
114 Wong ML, Kling MA, Munson PJ, Listwak S, Licinio J, Prolo P, Karp B, McCutcheon IE, Geracioti TD Jr., DeBellis MD, Rice KC, Goldstein DS, Veldhuis JD, Chrousos GP, Oldfield EH, McCann SM, Gold PW: Pronounced and sustained central hypernoradrenergic function in major depression with melancholic features: relation to hypercortisolism and corticotropin-releasing hormone. Proc Natl Acad Sci USA 2000;97:325–330.
115 Edwards AV: Regulation of adrenal function in the conscious calf. Horm Metab Res 1998;30:303–310.
116 Engeland WC: Functional innervation of the adrenal cortex by the splanchnic nerve. Horm Metab Res 1998;30:311–314.
117 Schmidt-Reinwald A, Pruessner JC, Hellhammer DH, Federenko I, Rohleder N, Schurmeyer TH, Kirschbaum C: The cortisol response to awakening in relation to different challenge tests and a 12-hour cortisol rhythm. Life Sci 1999;64:1653–1660.
118 Kirnap M, Colak R, Eser C, Ozsoy O, Tutus A, Kelestimur F: A comparison between low-dose (1 microg), standard-dose (250 microg) ACTH stimulation tests and insulin tolerance test in the evaluation of hypothalamo-pituitary-adrenal axis in primary fibromyalgia syndrome. Clin Endocrinol (Oxf) 2001;55:455–459.
119 Scott LV, Medbak S, Dinan TG: The low dose ACTH test in chronic fatigue syndrome and in health. Clin Endocrinol (Oxf) 1998;48:733–737.

120 DeRijk RH, Petrides J, Deuster P, Gold PW, Sternberg EM: Changes in corticosteroid sensitivity of peripheral blood lymphocytes after strenuous exercise in humans. J Clin Endocrinol Metab 1996; 81:228–235.
121 Yehuda R, Boisoneau D, Lowy MT, Giller EL Jr: Dose-response changes in plasma cortisol and lymphocyte glucocorticoid receptors following dexamethasone administration in combat veterans with and without posttraumatic stress disorder. Arch Gen Psychiatry 1995;52: 583–593.
122 McCormick JA, Lyons V, Jacobson MD, Noble J, Diorio J, Nyirenda M, Weaver S, Ester W, Yau JL, Meaney MJ, Seckl JR, Chapman KE: 5′-Heterogeneity of glucocorticoid receptor messenger RNA is tissue specific: differential regulation of variant transcripts by early-life events. Mol Endocrinol 2000;14:506–517.
123 Ebrecht M, Buske-Kirschbaum A, Hellhammer D, Kern S, Rohleder N, Walker B, Kirschbaum C: Tissue specificity of glucocorticoid sensitivity in healthy adults. J Clin Endocrinol Metab 2000;85: 3733–3739.
124 Dimitriadis G, Leighton B, Parry-Billings M, Sasson S, Young M, Krause U, Bevan S, Piva T, Wegener G, Newsholme EA: Effects of glucocorticoid excess on the sensitivity of glucose transport and metabolism to insulin in rat skeletal muscle. Biochem J 1997;321:707–712.
125 Pasquali R, Vicennati V: Activity of the hypothalamic-pituitary-adrenal axis in different obesity phenotypes. Int J Obes Relat Metab Disord 2000; 24(suppl 2):S47–S49.
126 Pasquali R, Vicennati V, Cacciari M, Pagotto U: The hypothalamic-pituitary-adrenal axis activity in obesity and the metabolic syndrome. Ann NY Acad Sci 2006;1083:111–128.
127 Young AH: Antiglucocoticoid treatments for depression. Aust NZ J Psychiatry 2006;40:402–405.
128 Belanoff JK, Rothschild AJ, Cassidy F, DeBattista C, Baulieu EE, Schold C, Schatzberg AF: An open label trial of C-1073 (mifepristone) for psychotic major depression. Biol Psychiatry 2002;52:386–392.
129 van Haarst AD, Oitzl MS, Workel JO, de Kloet ER: Chronic brain glucocorticoid receptor blockade enhances the rise in circadian and stress-induced pituitary-adrenal activity. Endocrinology 1996; 137:4935–4943.
130 Kirschbaum C, Wolf OT, May M, Wippich W, Hellhammer DH: Stress- and treatment-induced elevations of cortisol levels associated with impaired declarative memory in healthy adults. Life Sci 1996;58:1475–1483.
131 Wolf OT: HPA axis and memory. Best Pract Res Clin Endocrinol Metab 2003;17:287–299.
132 Lupien SJ, de Leon M, de Santi S, Convit A, Tarshish C, Nair NP, Thakur M, McEwen BS, Hauger RL, Meaney MJ: Cortisol levels during human aging predict hippocampal atrophy and memory deficits. Nat Neurosci 1998;1:69–73.
133 Lupien SJ, Lepage M: Stress, memory, and the hippocampus: can't live with it, can't live without it. Behav Brain Res 2001;127:137–158.
134 McEwen BS, de Leon MJ, Lupien SJ, Meaney MJ: Corticosteroids, the aging brain and cognition. Trends Endocrinol Metab 1999;10:92–96.

Hellhammer DH, Hellhammer J (eds): Stress. The Brain-Body Connection.
Key Issues in Mental Health. Basel, Karger, 2008, vol 174, pp 60–77

5. Hypocortisolemic Disorders

Eva Fries

Dysregulations of the hypothalamic-pituitary-adrenal axis (HPAA) are seen in several physical and psychiatric disorders and are discussed to be of major relevance for the symptoms reported by the respective patients. For example, a hyperactive HPAA was observed in melancholic depression, several anxiety disorders, diabetes type 2, hypertension or obesity [1]. In contrast, a hypoactive HPAA was described in irritable bowel syndrome, chronic pelvic pain, low back pain, burnout, fibromyalgia, rheumatoid arthritis, autoimmune diseases, chronic fatigue syndrome (CFS), post-traumatic stress disorder, and atypical depression [2]. Most hypocortisolism-associated disorders are characterized by symptoms of fatigue, pain and increased stress sensitivity, a constellation we recently termed 'hypocortisolemic symptom triad' [3].

As described in chapter 4, glucocorticoids (mainly cortisol in humans) – the end product of the HPAA – exert a wide range of action, inducing increased energy availability under acute stress [4]. Energy stores are mobilized via glucocorticoid-induced enhancement of gluconeogenesis und glycogenolysis and, additionally, via inhibition of glucose uptake in peripheral tissue. Furthermore, glucocorticoids act on lipid metabolism inducing an increased circulation of triglycerides and free fatty acids by lipolysis. Availability of amino acids for protein synthesis is influenced by glucocorticoids' actions on proteolysis. These effects of glucocorticoids all serve the need for increased energy demands during times of confrontation with a stressor [5].

Besides affecting energy availability, glucocorticoids furthermore act on the immune system suppressing, by distinct effects, pro-inflammatory mediators. For example, glucocorticoids inhibit inflammatory responses by suppressing the production and release of pro-inflammatory cytokines such as tumor necrosis factor-α (TNF-α), interleukin (IL)-1 and IL-6, cytokines known for orchestrating the early immune response to challenge by attracting and activating immune cells [6]. On the other hand, glucocorticoids stimulate anti-inflammatory mediators by enhancing the secretion of IL-4 or IL-10 by macrophages and Th2 cells and thus promoting Th2-

type immune reactions [7, 8]. The release of glucocorticoids during the acute stress response may thus restrain an inflammatory response to intruding pathogens as the immune reaction fighting these pathogens would weaken the organism in the acute stressful situation [7].

Furthermore, glucocorticoids released from the adrenal glands interact with another important stress response system, the sympathetic nervous system (SNS). The SNS constitutes one limb of the autonomic nervous system and its action is ergotropic, thus increasing the organism's ability to cope with a stressor. Nerve fibers of the SNS innervate several peripheral organs and the adrenal medulla, where the catecholamines epinephrine and norepinephrine are released at stimulation. In the periphery, glucocorticoids enhance myocardial contractility, contractility of blood vessels and baroreceptor sensitivity, but under acute stress they seem also to suppress catecholamine synthesis, turnover and release in sympathetic nerve fibers [9]. In the central nervous system, the locus coeruleus (LC), a nucleus with a dense network of noradrenergic cell bodies, has an important role in the regulation of the SNS. CRF enhances the unstimulated as well as the stress-induced activity of this nucleus [10], and increases the spontaneous discharge rate of LC neurons [11]. In contrast to CRF, peripheral released glucocorticoids act in an inhibitory fashion on the norepinephrine release in the central nervous system. For example, glucocorticoids inhibit the excitatory effects of CRF on noradrenergic neurons in the LC [12]. Thus, it seems that glucocorticoids have two actions on the ergotropic stress response: they facilitate SNS actions, but also dampen a noradrenergic overactivity in both the SNS and the central nervous system.

Glucocorticoids have a wide range of effects on bodily function, pointing to the importance of glucocorticoid release under acute stress conditions. However, at the time the organism is confronted with increased or decreased glucocorticoid levels for a prolonged period, glucocorticoids may have deleterious effects and, finally, several psychological and physical symptoms may emerge (see chapter 4). However, given the important role of glucocorticoids on bodily function, an intact HPAA is essential for psychological and physical health. A loss of glucocorticoid availability would thus create another spectrum of psychobiological symptoms. Indeed, Hellhammer and Wade [13] hypothesized a two-phase model, suggesting that chronic stress may first result in a prolonged hypercortisolism and, subsequently, in hypocortisolism. Under these conditions the adrenals remain enlarged but the production of cortisol is decreased [14, 15].

5.1. The Hypothalamic-Pituitary-Adrenal Axis in Hypocortisolemic Disorders

For several years, it was assumed that stress-related responses are characterized by an increased hyperactive HPAA, referred to as 'hypercortisolism' [1]. However, there is growing evidence that some subjects tend to develop a hypoactive HPAA when facing a period of several hours were measured in the cerebrospinal fluid of a small sample of depressed patients. At the same time, these patients displayed normal ACTH and cortisol levels [31]. Although levels of CRF in the cerebrospinal fluid are only an indirect marker of concentrations in the central nervous system, it is a feasible way to get access to neurotransmitters in the human brain. The pattern of low CRF levels in cerebrospinal fluid with normal cortisol levels was confirmed in a subsequent study on depressed in-patients of whom the majority had a least one 'atypical symptom', such as hypersomnia and hypoarousal, hyperphagia, or loss of energy [32].

Description of symptoms associated with atypical depression shows the proximity of different hypocortisolemic disorders as well as a great symptom overlap and comorbidity among distinct clinical entities [33]. For example, fatigue and hypoarousal are not only expressed in atypical depression, but are core symptoms of CFS, where a CRF hypoactivity was described in a subgroup of patients [34]. Another clinical condition, which is likewise characterized by symptoms of fatigue, hypoarousal, hyperphagia or loss of energy, is Cushing's disease. Again, for this clinical entity results exist pointing towards reduced CRF activity in the brain [35]. Cushing's disease is a pathological condition with very high cortisol levels, which block CRF synthesis and release via the negative feedback loop. An abnormal ACTH and cortisol response to ovine CRF stimulation, as an indicator of hypofunctioning CRF neurons, was also reported in patients with seasonal affective disorders [36], again a clinical entity showing great symptom overlap with atypical depression. Due to the wide overlap of symptoms and biological correlates between atypical depression, CFS and other disorders, it is suggested that biological mechanisms rather than clinical diagnoses have to be considered in appropriate diagnostic and therapeutic treatments [33, 37].

Focusing on the role of CRF in the regulation of arousal and sleep, the strong innervation of the LC, the major noradrenergic nucleus in the brain stem, is of relevance [38]. For example, CRF enhances the unstimulated as well as the stress-induced activity of this nucleus [10] and increases the spontaneous discharge rate of LC neurons [11]. From the LC, noradrenergic fibers project to numerous brain regions increasing arousal, attention and vigilance [39]. At the same time, the PVN of the hypothalamus is strongly innervated by noradrenergic neurons from the LC, thus depicting a positive feedback loop between PVN and LC [38]. Due to this close interaction (among other mechanisms), sufficient CRF seems to be necessary for evoking and maintaining arousal, particularly under conditions which need CRF activation for the adaptation to stress.

Considering the central role of CRF in the coordination of the stress response and the modulatory influence on cognition, mood and arousal, a relative lack of CRF may thus have extensive consequences, e.g. hypoarousal and hypersomnia. Whereas increased activity of CRF in the central nervous system was linked with hyperarousal and insomnia [40], there is evidence – as described above – linking decreased CRF activity with hypoarousal and hypersomnia in different diagnostic categories.

The above-described picture of CRF hypoactivity with symptoms of hypoarousal and hypersomnia is in contrast to one of the core symptoms of the 'hypocortisolemic symptom triad': increased stress sensitivity. The underlying mechanism of increased stress sensitivity, as seen for example in PTSD, may be reduced glucocorticoid signaling and negative feedback to the central nervous system, resulting in disinhibition of CRF and norepinephrine. This is supported by studies showing reduced cortisol levels in PTSD patients with, at the same time, indicators of increased CRF reactivity [41].

Further, even a hyporesponsivity of the pituitary may account for a hypocortisolemic stress response. In patients with atopic disorders with no signs of (atypical) depression or major psychological stress, a blunted ACTH response has been observed after both CRF challenge [42] and psychological stress [43].

5.2.2. Cortisol Hypoactivity

Alterations of the HPAA at the peripheral level seem, for example, to be of importance in fatigue and exhaustion: numerous observations showed a decreased HPAA activity in CFS with fatigue as the core symptom. Considering the daily variation in cortisol secretion in CFS patients, a diminished cortisol rise after awakening [22], and reduced cortisol levels during the day were observed [34, 44–46]. Additionally, an increased negative feedback sensitivity of the HPAA, as indicated by an enhanced and prolonged cortisol suppression after dexamethasone intake, was described in several studies [46, 47]. However, conflicting results do exist [34, 48, 49]. The relevance of cortisol for the subjective feeling of fatigue is underscored by results showing an improvement of fatigue after therapy with hydrocortisone in healthy subjects [50] and patients with CFS [51, 52].

In parallel to the observations in CFS, numerous studies also point towards a hypoactive HPAA in major depression with atypical features [20, 53]. An increased negative feedback sensitivity of the HPAA, indicated by a greater suppression of endogenous cortisol in the low-dose dexamethasone suppression test, was observed in depressed women with atypical features [54]. The importance of a relative lack of cortisol for the symptomatology in depression with atypical features is underlined by preliminary findings showing an improvement in depressive symptoms after prednisone [55] or dexamethasone therapy [56].

Considering the importance of hypocortisolism for the experience of fatigue, exhaustion, and behavioral depression as observed in CFS or atypical depression, the concept of 'sickness behavior' may explain underlying mechanisms of the symptoms. Typical symptoms of sickness behavior are malaise, lassitude, fatigue, numbness, coldness as well as muscle and joint aches, some of the symptoms also characterizing CFS or atypical depression. Sickness behavior is triggered by pro-inflammatory cytokines acting via neural and humoral pathways on the central nervous system [57]. Considering the neural signaling route, the vagus nerve plays an important role as sensory neurons of the vagus nerve express receptors for pro-inflammatory cytokines. At cytokine binding at the respective receptors, the nerve fibers of the vagus send afferent information to the central nervous system and thereby induce some symptoms of sickness behavior, especially behavioral depression. Additionally, the glossopharyngeal nerves have been identified to relay information about inflammation or infection from the periphery to the brain. On the humoral route, intermediate mediators transport the signals from the peripheral immune system to the brain. These molecular intermediates, mainly prostaglandins of the class E_2, are produced at the level of blood-brain interfaces in response to circulating cytokines. Prostaglandins then diffuse into different brain areas and induce the sickness behavior. In addition to behavioral effects, the HPAA is activated during the acute sickness response. However, it may be speculated that the HPAA downregulates at continuation of the sickness response. Nevertheless, the acute sickness behavior, characterized by fatigue and behavioral depression among others, may be adaptive in favor of a reorganization of the priorities of the host during an infectious episode, thus promoting subsequent recuperation [review in 6, 57].

Despite the relevance of the acute sickness response, a prolonged and inadequate sickness response has been discussed to play a role in the symptoms of CFS and atypical depression [28]. As described above, glucocorticoids have profound suppressive effects on pro-inflammatory cytokines such as IL-1 or IL-6 [7]. In the case of reduced, 'hypocortisolemic' cortisol levels, as seen in the patient described below, the suppressive effects of cortisol on pro-inflammatory mediators may be reduced and thus promote increased pro-inflammatory cytokines with enhanced signaling to the central nervous system, finally resulting in pronounced sickness behavior with the symptoms described above. This hypothesis is in line with evidence showing an enhanced immune status in patients with severe fatigue symptomatology; for example, elevated levels of pro-inflammatory cytokines have been described in patients with CFS [58]. Also, a role of dysfunctions of the immune system has been proposed for the symptoms seen in atypical depression [28].

Case Report

A 47-year-old male organ maker presented with major impairments of physical and psychological well-being. As his currently most overriding symptoms, he described burnout and musculoskeletal pain. He described himself as being mostly unable to initiate activity and as being completely exhausted, even after mild physical exercise. Also, he felt mentally exhausted due to permanent job demands and described feelings of being physically powerless and weak. He compared his physical status to the symptoms of having the flu with feelings of malaise, lassitude, fatigue, numbness and coldness. He further reported increasing restlessness, uneasiness, irritability, and excitability, creating increasing tension in his partnership and social environment.

The patient reported that the onset of his symptoms occurred after a period of intense, prolonged stress. He had to build three new organs in a period of 7 months, and was spending about 12–16 h in his shop during that time. After finishing his work in time, he first developed mental fatigue, then irritability, and finally musculoskeletal pain. Within the next 3 months he felt almost unable to continue his job, which created financial problems since he was self-employed.

When neuropattern was applied, he fulfilled the criteria for 'cortisol hypoactivity'. His cortisol levels at awakening were very low (2.7 nmol/l) with a subsequent increase of 9.2 nmol/l. During the day, his cortisol levels remained in the lower range, and he showed a pronounced suppression of cortisol levels after taking dexamethasone. He expressed typical symptoms of the hypocortisolism triad, as described above.

The period of intense stress has been accompanied by anticipatory worrying, ego involvement and unpredictability, suggesting a prolonged activation of the HPAA. After successfully finishing his work, a subsequent hypocortisolemic period may have developed, as verified by low cortisol levels and supersuppression of cortisol after dexamethasone intake. The concomitant onset of fatigue, pain, and uneasiness may have been caused by disinhibition of pro-inflammatory cytokines and/or prostaglandins as described above. Evidence for such effects of chronic stress was recently provided by Kiecolt-Glaser* who reported that caregivers' average rate of increase in IL-6 was about four times as high as that of noncaregivers.

* Kiecolt-Glaser JK, Preacher KJ, MacCallum RC, Atkinson C, Malarkey WB, Glaser R: Chronic stress and age-related increases in the proinflammatory cytokine IL-6. Proc Natl Acad Sci US A 2003;100:9090–9095.

Increased pain sensitivity has also been ascribed to symptoms of the 'hypocortisolemic symptom triad' [3] and is most often seen in patients with fibromyalgia. However, pain is also reported by patients with a diagnosis of CFS [59] or PTSD [60], thus illustrating the symptom overlap between distinct diagnostic categories. Fibromyalgia, a prominent disorder for the 'hypocortisolemic symptom triad' is characterized by the core symptoms of widespread, chronic musculoskeletal pain, pressure hyperalgesia and, additionally, by alterations in HPAA functioning. Considering adrenal cortisol, reduced concentrations of glucocorticoids were detected in 24-hour urine samples of patients with fibromyalgia [17, 61, 62], although normal glucocorticoid concentrations in 24-hour urine samples were described in some studies [63–65]. A normal cortisol response was seen in most studies, applying low-to-normal synacthen challenges [17, 64]. Additionally, increased negative feedback sensitivity, indicated by an increased and prolonged cortisol suppression in the low-dose dexamethasone suppression test, was reported in patients with chronic pain [66]. Concluding, robust findings in fibromyalgia are reduced cortisol levels during the day, thus possibly linking reduced cortisol levels to the core symptom of fibromyalgia, namely pain. The association between reduced cortisol levels and increased pain perception is further underlined by findings of low cortisol levels in other disorders characterized by pain sensation such as low back pain [67], chronic pelvic pain [18], or irritable bowel syndrome [68].

A recent study by Klingmann et al. [69] suggests that this type of cortisol hypoactivity may already be programmed in the prenatal period. In this study, neuropattern was applied in 93 female and 10 male patients with fibromyalgia. The authors reported that most of the female patients fulfilled the criteria for cortisol hypoactivity and showed a blunted cortisol response to awakening. Considering the patients' case history, it became obvious that the blunted cortisol response to awakening was only observed in those 60% of female patients reporting short gestational length. This suggests possible prenatal programming of adrenal capacity. The authors assumed that the prenatal programming of reduced adrenal capacity may constitute a vulnerability factor, since insufficient amounts of cortisol may be released from the adrenals at confrontation with major stressors in later life. Consequently, these subjects may be unable to buffer the massive increase of pro-inflammatory cytokines, mobilized under psychological or physical major stress. The authors propose the manifestation of a fatigue and pain memory under such conditions.

As a recent study showed, prenatal stress results in an altered stress responsivity in later life with clear gender differences: while men show both an enhanced ACTH and cortisol response to psychosocial stress, women emit an enhanced ACTH response, but, surprisingly, a blunted cortisol response [70, 71]. These studies provide further evidence on gender-specific prenatal programming.

As another important link between reduced cortisol concentrations and pain symptomatology, one may consider the effects of glucocorticoids on prostaglandins. Converted from arachnidonic acid by cyclo-oxygenases COX-1 and COX-2, prostaglandins are important mediators of pain perception. They sensitize the nociceptive system at the level of peripheral receptors located on the peripheral terminal of primary sensory neurons resulting in enhanced perception of pain. In addition to their peripheral effect, peripherally released prostaglandins also exert effects on the central nervous system, mainly at the level of the spinal cord. Here, prostaglandins seem to sensitize specific nociceptive pathways leading to central or secondary hyperalgesia, a state of increased pain sensitivity. Additionally, centrally acting prostagladins elicit mechanical allodynia resulting in pain perception at stimulation of low-threshold mechanosensitive fibers [72]. Synthetic glucocorticoids are prominent drugs in the therapy of inflammation [73] as well as in pain [74]. This efficacy of glucocorticoids in the treatment of inflammation and pain may partly be ascribed to the suppressive effects of endogenous and exogenous glucocorticoids on the prostaglandin synthesis via inhibition of COX-2 [75].

Coming back to the 'hypocortisolemic symptom triad', as described above, prostaglandins participate in elicitation of the sickness response characterized by elevated body temperature, altered mood and fatigue [72] and, additionally, by sickness-induced pain facilitation [6]. In sickness-induced pain facilitation, prostaglandins and cytokines seem to act on microglia at the level of the spinal cord which subsequently leads to hyperexitability of the pain transmission neurons. This hyperexcitability may then result in maintenance of the pain symptomatology. However, sickness-induced pain facilitation may also occur at the level of the peripheral nerves, dorsal root ganglia or at higher brain areas [6, 76].

Summarizing the role of glucocorticoids in the symptomatology of pain, the suppressive effects of glucocorticoids on the synthesis of prostaglandins and pro-inflammatory cytokines both modulate the pain and the sickness response. It is thus likely that even a mild hypocortisolism may contribute substantially to the symptom of enhanced pain sensitivity as seen in several hypocortisolemic disorders.

This short description of underlying mechanisms of different 'hypocortisolemic' symptoms demonstrates how divergent symptoms develop depending on the level of HPAA disturbances. It further underlines the striking need for detailed diagnostics in patients with hypocortisolemic disorders taking the different levels of the HPAA into consideration. The level of hypocortisolemic dysfunction can be discriminated once suitable measures are taken.

5.3. Conceptualization of Hypocortisolism

As already described, one may speculate that hypoactivity at one or more levels of the HPAA may causally be related to the experience of pronounced fatigue, hypoarousal, hypersomnia and increased pain sensitivity as seen for example in the patient described in 'Case Report'.

As mentioned above, chronic stress and several stress-related disorders are characterized by an increased, hyperactive HPAA [1]. However, some subjects develop a hypoactive HPAA when facing chronic or traumatic stress. It is not yet fully elucidated why some subjects develop a hypoactive and others a hyperactive HPAA. Hellhammer and Wade [13] postulated that a hypoactive HPAA may result after prolonged periods of chronic or traumatic stress, which may at first be accompanied by enhanced HPAA activity resulting in increased cortisol secretion from the adrenal glands. The increased HPAA activity may serve to improve the organism's functioning in the face of current stressors. However, at continuation of chronic stress, a hypoactive HPAA may develop, whereas the switch in HPAA activity may be ascribed to the self-adjusting abilities of the organism with the objective of protecting the organism against the possible deleterious effects of chronic high glucocorticoid exposure. In the case of the development of hypocortisolism, one may assume a failure in the organism's self-adjusting abilities, resulting in an 'over-adjustment' and, thus, in a hypoactive HPAA [2, 3].

Possible mechanisms of HPAA adjustment are (1) downregulation of specific receptors at different levels of the axis (hypothalamus, pituitary, adrenals, target cells), (2) reduced biosynthesis or depletion at several levels of the HPAA (CRF, ACTH, cortisol), and/or (3) increased negative feedback sensitivity to glucocorticoids [2, 3, 13]. This model for the development of hypocortisolism is supported by a recent meta-analysis conducted by Miller et al. [77] which analyzed publications under the viewpoint of the association of time since stressor occurrence (e.g. combat/war experience, abuse/assault, death/loss of a major relationship, care-giving experience, natural disaster, job loss/unemployment) to alteration of HPAA activity. One of the most robust findings of the meta-analysis was a negative association between time since onset of the stressor and HPAA activity, thus supporting the model of an initial activation of the HPAA followed by a diminished HPAA activity with time passing by.

Our conceptualization of hypocortisolism is additionally underlined by recent evidence from animal experiments. Houshyar et al. [78–80] exposed rats to chronic (16 days) morphine treatment, whereas the emerging morphine dependence may be considered as a chronic stressor. In line with the above-stated model for the development of a hypoactive HPAA, the rats first showed increased HPAA activity as well as prolonged and elevated ACTH and glucocorticoid levels at discontinuation of morphine treatment. However, 8 days after the termination of morphine treatment, the animals displayed HPAA characteristics specific to hypocortisolism: despite normal-to-reduced ACTH levels and normal glucocorticoid levels under basal, unstimulated conditions, animals showed blunted ACTH and reduced (to normal) glucocorticoid response to an acute restraint stress [78–80]. When dexamethasone (max. 1 mg/kg s.c.) was administered to these animals prior to stress exposure, the animals displayed a markedly reduced ACTH response to restraint stress ('super-suppression') compared to similarly treated nondependent animals. However, glucocorticoid response to restraint stress was normally suppressed and, additionally, ACTH and glucocorticoid secretion in response to CRF stimulation was normal, thus demonstrating an increased sensitivity to glucocorticoid negative feedback at the level of the pituitary and no changes of CRF receptors at the level of the pituitary [79]. These results support the above-stated model for the development of a hypoactive HPAA, showing that chronic stress eventually results in a hypoactivity.

Additionally, dispositional factors such as genetic or developmental factors may account for an increased vulnerability for the development of a hypoactive HPAA and hypocortisolemic symptoms. Whereas no direct studies on the genetic transmission of hypocortisolism exist, evidence indicates a genetic influence on HPAA functioning in general [81–83]. Also, for several disorders characterized by hypocortisolism, a genetic contribution and an increased accumulation within families was observed [84, 85], additionally suggesting a possible genetic basis for hypocortisolemic symptoms. A prominent contribution to a hypoactive HPAA may also come from variations in the genetic code (e.g. selective nuclear polymorphisms) which, for example, may account for reduced cortisol synthesis due to enzyme deficits [86], increased cortisol availability in the central nervous system with an increased negative feedback regulation of the HPAA due to a reduced number of multi-drug resistance gene 1-type P-glycoproteins [87], or changed glucocorticoid receptor status and, thus, enhanced negative feedback sensitivity [88].

In addition to or in interaction with genetic factors, developmental factors may play a pivotal role in shaping HPAA functioning. Especially the prenatal period seems to be of major importance in the 'programming' of later HPAA functioning [review in 89], also with respect to a hypocortisolemic HPAA (see also above). The maternal HPAA seems to be an important mediator of environmental effects (e.g. maternal stress, infection) on the fetus: in animals, high maternal glucocorticoids during pregnancy were associated with adrenal hypotrophy and a reduced stress-induced HPAA activation in the (female) adult offspring [90]. Additionally, prenatal factors such as malnutrition or hypoxia are associated with reduced cortisol levels, increased negative feedback sensitivity of the HPAA [91, 92] and reduced adrenal sensitivity to ACTH stimulation [93], respectively. Interestingly, Yehuda et al. [94] showed that severe psychological stress in pregnant women (such as experienced during the 2001 attacks on the World Trade Center) was associated with lower cortisol levels in babies of mothers developing PTSD compared to babies of mothers not developing PTSD. This shows that different factors emerge during pregnancy and impact on the developing HPAA of the fetus, thus making it more vulnerable for the development of a hypoactive HPAA.

In addition to prenatal programming, postnatal factors such as early life events or perceived maternal care are of relevance for HPAA functioning, predominantly shown in animal studies [95]. However, also human studies provide evidence for this association: for example, sexually abused girls showed a reduced ACTH secretion, but normal cortisol secretion in response to stimulation with CRF [96]. In adult women, a blunted adrenal response to ACTH stimulation was observed in women who were sexually abused during childhood [97]. The same pattern of ACTH and cortisol response to CRF stimulation was seen in adult women with current PTSD after early childhood sexual abuse. Additionally, these women displayed lower afternoon cortisol levels when compared with healthy controls [98]. Thus, these results show an altered HPAA activation after early adverse life events in the direction of a hypocortisolemic status, and may enhance vulnerability for hypocortisolemic disorders such as CFS [99].

5.4. Protective Effects of Hypocortisolism

As cortisol has numerous and extensive effects on physiological and psychological functions, the relative lack of cortisol seen in hypocortisolism seems to be associated with several symptoms (see above, 'hypocortisolemic symptom triad'). However, despite the profound costs of hypocortisolism, the development of a hypoactive HPAA may also have protective consequences for the organism.

One line of evidence towards the protective effects of hypocortisolism refers to the concept of 'allostatic load', first introduced by McEwen and Stellar [100]. This concept describes the wear and tear of the body and brain resulting from chronic hyperactivity or inactivation of physiological systems that are normally involved in adaptation to environmental challenges. High allostatic load results when the allostatic systems are either overworked or fail to shut off after the stressful event or when these systems fail to respond adequately to the initial challenge, leading other systems to overreact [101]. However, Hellhammer et al. [102] challenged this concept, demonstrating the coexistence of high stress but low allostatic load in hypocortisolemic subjects. The authors hypothesized that hypocortisolism may have protective effects for some but not all stress-related disorders. In line with their results, Raison and Miller [103] argued that hypocortisolism may be caused by prolonged or repeated exposure to immune stimuli in the sense of freeing bodily defenses from the inhibitory control of glucocorticoids. As a result, increased release of inflammatory mediators may be adaptive in conditions of recurrent, threatening infection, thus increasing immune readiness at confrontation with relevant stimuli.

Concluding, a hypoactive HPAA with reduced cortisol secretion is not only maladaptive but may even have beneficial effects for the organism's survival. For example, low cortisol levels in subjects continuously or repeatedly exposed to immune stimuli facilitate a rapid combat of immune stimuli. Interestingly, a low allostatic load in hypocortisolemic subjects suggests that downregulation of HPAA activity may be protective against deleterious effects of chronic glucocorticoid overexposure and, thus, high allostatic load. However, protective and beneficial effects of hypocortisolism for the organism pay the cost by having symptoms such as fatigue, pain and enhanced stress sensitivity.

5.5. Conclusions

For a long time, research on the glandotropic stress response has exclusively focused on hypercortisolism. However, in the last two decades, it became increasingly evident that probably most so-called 'psychosomatic' disorders are rather characterized by hypocortisolism. Today, one can discriminate the origin of hypocortisolemic disorders at the levels of the hypothalamus, the pituitary, the adrenals, and receptor sites. The neuropattern approach allows a first screening and generates tentative diagnoses for further differential diagnostic and therapeutic treatments. The case described above illustrates a typical feature of a hypocortisolemic patient. Our diagnosis did not support alternative explanations of his burnout symptomatology, since he did not qualify for other neuropatterns such as CRF hypoactivity, serotonin hyperactivity, and norepinephrine depletion. The report informed the physician about our tentative diagnosis and possible differential diagnostic treatments needed to control our assumptions. The report further included concrete treatment recommendations.

5.6. Summary

Despite increasing knowledge on HPAA dysfunction in different disorders, at the moment, the findings are only of minor relevance in the explanation and treatment of patients with the respective symptoms. Therefore, the present chapter makes attempts to discuss the possible relevance of HPAA hypoactivity for symptoms of the 'hypocortisolemic symptom triad'. In this context, potentially underlying physiological mechanisms linking HPAA hypoactivity at a central or peripheral level with, for example, hypoarousal, hypersomnia, pain, or fatigue, are addressed. Additionally, a hypothetical model on the development of a hypoactive HPAA is provided and the possible protective effects of hypocortisolism are discussed. Finally, a case report of a male patient presenting with symptoms of apathy, listlessness, tiredness, fatigue, and pain is given.

References

1 Chrousos GP, Gold PW: The concepts of stress and stress system disorders: overview of physical and behavioral homeostasis. JAMA 1992;267:1244–1252.

2 Heim C, Ehlert U, Hellhammer DH: The potential role of hypocortisolism in the pathophysiology of stress-related bodily disorders. Psychoneuroendocrinology 2000;25:1–35.

3 Fries E, Hesse J, Hellhammer J, Hellhammer DH: A new view on hypocortisolism. Psychoneuroendocrinology 2005;30:1010–1016.

4 Pacak K, McCarty R: Acute stress response: experimental; in Fink G (ed): Encyclopedia of Stress. San Diego, Academic Press, 2000, pp 8–17.

5 Murphy BEP: Glucocorticoids, Overview; in Fink G (ed): Encyclopedia of Stress. San Diego, Academic Press, 2000, pp 244–261.

6 Watkins LR, Maier SF: Immune regulation of central nervous system functions: from sickness responses to pathological pain. J Intern Med 2005;257:139–155.

7 Franchimont D, Kino T, Galon J, Meduri GU, Chrousos G: Glucocorticoids and inflammation revisited: the state of the art: NIH clinical staff conference. Neuroimmunomodulation 2002;10:247–260.

8 Ramirez F, Fowell DJ, Puklavec M, Simmonds S, Mason D: Glucocorticoids promote a TH2 cytokine response by CD4+ T cells in vitro. J Immunol 1996;156:2406–2412.

9 Kvetnansky R, Fukuhara K, Pacak K, Cizza G, Goldstein DS, Kopin IJ: Endogenous glucocorticoids restrain catecholamine synthesis and release at rest and during immobilization stress in rats. Endocrinology 1993;133:1411–1419.

10 Valentino RJ, Page ME, Curtis AL: Activation of noradrenergic locus coeruleus neurons by hemodynamic stress is due to local release of corticotropin-releasing factor. Brain Res 1991;555:25–34.

11 Valentino RJ: CRH effects on central noradrenergic neurons: relationship to stress. Adv Exp Med Biol 1988;245:47–64.

12 Lechner SM, Valentino RJ: Glucocorticoid receptor-immunoreactivity in corticotrophin-releasing factor afferents to the locus coeruleus. Brain Res 1999;816:17–28.

13 Hellhammer DH, Wade S: Endocrine correlates of stress vulnerability. Psychother Psychosom 1993;60:8–17.

14 Reber SO, Birkeneder L, Veenema AH, Obermeier F, Falk W, Straub RH, Neumann ID: Adrenal insufficiency and colonic inflammation after a novel chronic psycho-social stress paradigm in mice: implications and mechanisms. Endocrinology 2007;148:670–682.

15 Reber SO, Obermeier F, Straub RH, Falk W, Neumann ID: Chronic intermittent psychosocial stress (social defeat/overcrowding) in mice increases the severity of an acute DSS-induced colitis and impairs regeneration. Endocrinology 2006;147:4968–4976.

16 Yehuda R, Giller EL, Southwick SM, Lowy MT, Mason JW: Hypothalamic-pituitary-adrenal dysfunction in posttraumatic stress disorder. Biol Psychiatry 1991;30:1031–1048.

17 Griep EN, Boersma JW, Lentjes EG, Prins AP, van der Korst JK, de Kloet ER: Function of the hypothalamic-pituitary-adrenal axis in patients with fibromyalgia and low back pain. J Rheumatol 1998;25:1374–1381.

18 Heim C, Ehlert U, Hanker JP, Hellhammer DH: Abuse-related posttraumatic stress disorder and alterations of the hypothalamic-pituitary-adrenal axis in women with chronic pelvic pain. Psychosom Med 1998;60:309–318.

19 Pruessner JC, Hellhammer DH, Kirschbaum C: Burnout, perceived stress, and cortisol responses to awakening. Psychosom Med 1999;61:197–204.

20 Gold PW, Chrousos GP: Organization of the stress system and its dysregulation in melancholic and atypical depression: high vs. low CRH/NE states. Mol Psychiatry 2002;7:254–275.

21 Gur A, Cevik R, Nas K, Colpan L, Sarac S: Cortisol and hypothalamic-pituitary-gonadal axis hormones in follicular-phase women with fibromyalgia and chronic fatigue syndrome and effect of depressive symptoms on these hormones. Arthritis Res Ther 2004;6:R232–R238.

22 Roberts AD, Wessely S, Chalder T, Papadopoulos A, Cleare AJ: Salivary cortisol response to awakening in chronic fatigue syndrome. Br J Psychiatry 2004;184:136–141.

23 Rohleder N, Joksimovic L, Wolf JM, Kirschbaum C: Hypocortisolism and increased glucocorticoid sensitivity of pro-inflammatory cytokine production in Bosnian war refugees with posttraumatic stress disorder. Biol Psychiatry 2004;55:745–751.

24 Rohleder N, Wolf JM, Kirschbaum C: Glucocorticoid sensitivity in humans-interindividual differences and acute stress effects. Stress 2003;6:207–222.

25 Chrousos GP, Kino T: Glucocorticoid action networks and complex psychiatric and/or somatic disorders. Stress 2007;10:213–219.

26 Ford JD, Campbell KA, Storzbach D, Binder LM, Anger WK, Rohlman DS: Posttraumatic stress symptomatology is associated with unexplained illness attributed to Persian Gulf War military service. Psychosom Med 2001;63:842–849.

77 Miller GE, Chen E, Zhou ES: If it goes up, must it come down? Chronic stress and the hypothalamic-pituitary-adrenocortical axis in humans. Psychol Bull 2007;133:25–45.
78 Houshyar H, Cooper ZD, Woods JH: Paradoxical effects of chronic morphine treatment on the temperature and pituitary-adrenal responses to acute restraint stress: a chronic stress paradigm. J Neuroendocrinol 2001;13:862–874.
79 Houshyar H, Galigniana MD, Pratt WB, Woods JH: Differential responsivity of the hypothalamic-pituitary-adrenal axis to glucocorticoid negative-feedback and corticotropin releasing hormone in rats undergoing morphine withdrawal: possible mechanisms involved in facilitated and attenuated stress responses. J Neuroendocrinol 2001;13:875–886.
80 Houshyar H, Gomez F, Manalo S, Bhargava A, Dallman MF: Intermittent morphine administration induces dependence and is a chronic stressor in rats. Neuropsychopharmacology 2003;28:1960–1972.
81 Wust S, Federenko IS, van Rossum EF, Koper JW, Hellhammer DH: Habituation of cortisol responses to repeated psychosocial stress-further characterization and impact of genetic factors. Psychoneuroendocrinology 2005;30:199–211.
82 Kirschbaum C, Wust S, Faig HG, Hellhammer DH: Heritability of cortisol responses to human corticotropin-releasing hormone, ergometry, and psychological stress in humans. J Clin Endocrinol Metab 1992;75:1526–1530.
83 Wust S, Federenko I, Hellhammer DH, Kirschbaum C: Genetic factors, perceived chronic stress, and the free cortisol response to awakening. Psychoneuroendocrinology 2000;25:707–720.
84 Segman RH, Shalev AY: Genetics of posttraumatic stress disorder. CNS Spectr 2003;8:693–698.
85 Arnold LM, Hudson JI, Hess EV, Ware AE, Fritz DA, Auchenbach MB, Starck LO, Keck PE Jr: Family study of fibromyalgia. Arthritis Rheum 2004;50:944–952.
86 Charmandari E, Merke DP, Negro PJ, Keil MF, Martinez PE, Haim A, Gold PW, Chrousos GP: Endocrinologic and psychologic evaluation of 21-hydroxylase deficiency carriers and matched normal subjects: evidence for physical and/or psychologic vulnerability to stress. J Clin Endocrinol Metab 2004;89:2228–2236.
87 Muller MB, Keck ME, Binder EB, Kresse AE, Hagemeyer TP, Landgraf R, Holsboer F, Uhr M: ABCB1 (MDR1)-type P-glycoproteins at the blood-brain barrier modulate the activity of the hypothalamic-pituitary-adrenocortical system: implications for affective disorder. Neuropsychopharmacology 2003;28:1991–1999.
88 Wust S, Van Rossum EF, Federenko IS, Koper JW, Kumsta R, Hellhammer DH: Common polymorphisms in the glucocorticoid receptor gene are associated with adrenocortical responses to psychosocial stress. J Clin Endocrinol Metab 2004;89:565–573.
89 Welberg LA, Seckl JR, Holmes MC: Prenatal glucocorticoid programming of brain corticosteroid receptors and corticotrophin-releasing hormone: possible implications for behaviour. Neuroscience 2001;104:71–79.
90 Fameli M, Kitraki E, Stylianopoulou F: Effects of hyperactivity of the maternal hypothalamic-pituitary-adrenal (HPA) axis during pregnancy on the development of the HPA axis and brain monoamines of the offspring. Int J Dev Neurosci 1994;12:651–659.
91 Kajantie E, Phillips DI, Andersson S, Barker DJ, Dunkel L, Forsen T, Osmond C, Tuominen J, Wood PJ, Eriksson J: Size at birth, gestational age and cortisol secretion in adult life: foetal programming of both hyper- and hypocortisolism? Clin Endocrinol (Oxf) 2002;57:635–641.
92 Kajantie E, Eriksson J, Barker DJ, Forsen T, Osmond C, Wood PJ, Andersson S, Dunkel L, Phillips DI: Birthsize, gestational age and adrenal function in adult life: studies of dexamethasone suppression and ACTH1-24 stimulation. Eur J Endocrinol 2003;149:569–575.
93 Ducsay CA: Fetal and maternal adaptations to chronic hypoxia: prevention of premature labor in response to chronic stress. Comp Biochem Physiol [A] 1998;119:675–681.
94 Yehuda R, Engel SM, Brand SR, Seckl J, Marcus SM, Berkowitz GS: Transgenerational effects of posttraumatic stress disorder in babies of mothers exposed to the World Trade Center attacks during pregnancy. J Clin Endocrinol Metab 2005;90:4115–4118.
95 Meaney MJ: Maternal care, gene expression, and the transmission of individual differences in stress reactivity across generations. Ann Rev Neurosci 2001;24:1161–1192.
96 De Bellis MD, Chrousos GP, Dorn LD, Burke L, Helmers K, Kling MA, Trickett PK, Putnam FW: Hypothalamic-pituitary-adrenal axis dysregulation in sexually abused girls. J Clin Endocrinol Metab 1994;78:249–255.
97 Heim C, Newport DJ, Bonsall R, Miller AH, Nemeroff CB: Altered pituitary-adrenal axis responses to provocative challenge tests in adult survivors of childhood abuse. Am J Psychiatry 2001;158:575–581.

98 Bremner JD, Vythilingam M, Anderson G, Vermetten E, McGlashan T, Heninger G, Rasmusson A, Southwick SM, Charney DS: Assessment of the hypothalamic-pituitary-adrenal axis over a 24-hour diurnal period and in response to neuroendocrine challenges in women with and without childhood sexual abuse and posttraumatic stress disorder. Biol Psychiatry 2003;54:710–718.
99 Heim C, Wagner D, Maloney E, Papanicolaou DA, Solomon L, Jones JF, Unger ER, Reeves WC: Early adverse experience and risk for chronic fatigue syndrome: results from a population-based study. Arch Gen Psychiatry 2006;63:1258–1266.
100 McEwen BS, Stellar E: Stress and the individual: mechanisms leading to disease. Arch Intern Med 1993;153:2093–2101.
101 McEwen BS, Wingfield JC: The concept of allostasis in biology and biomedicine. Horm Behav 2003; 43:2–15.
102 Hellhammer J, Schlotz W, Stone AA, Pirke KM, Hellhammer D: Allostatic load, perceived stress, and health: a prospective study in two age groups. Ann NY Acad Sci 2004;1032:8–13.
103 Raison CL, Miller AH: When not enough is too much: the role of insufficient glucocorticoid signaling in the pathophysiology of stress-related disorders. Am J Psychiatry 2003;160:1554–1565.

Hellhammer DH, Hellhammer J (eds): Stress. The Brain-Body Connection.
Key Issues in Mental Health. Basel, Karger, 2008, vol 174, pp 78–90

6. Noradrenergic and Sympathetic Disorders

Pascal O. Klingmann • Dirk H. Hellhammer

As introduced in chapter 3, an ergotropic state of the organism is characterized by active adaptation to demands such as physical or mental work, or under stress conditions. Two systems mainly control ergotropic states, the dorsal noradrenergic bundle, originating from the locus coeruleus (LC) in the brain stem, and the sympathetic nervous system (SNS). The functional synergism of both ergotropic systems is mainly integrated and controlled by the paraventricular nucleus of the hypothalamus (PVN), as described in chapter 3. This seems to be necessary, given the importance of the SNS in regulating organ function. The stress response should always be integrated into the current physiological state, and the PVN is the integrator by receiving such visceral and endocrine signals from both the brain and the periphery [1]. Central noradrenergic neurons per se facilitate alertness and attention to environmental stimuli, while the SNS controls the peripheral organs for a most efficient adaptation for physical work, fight and flight by increasing heart rate and breathing, constricting blood vessels, releasing glucose, tightening muscles, and activating the immune system.

In this chapter, we will address mental and physical disorders which are, at least in part, affected by ergotropic systems. We will then try to characterize the role of different ergotropic endophenotypes in these types of health disturbances by their respective psychological, biological and symptomatic features.

6.1. Determinants of Ergotropy

Both the dorsal noradrenergic and the SNS contribute considerably to stress effects on mental and physical disorders. However, it seems that both ergotropic systems affect the magnitude rather than the quality of the expression of a given symptom. This, however, may strongly determine the vulnerability for and the maintenance of such symptoms. It is not surprising that the spectrum of stress-related disorders seems to be linked phylogenetically to fight and flight behavior: for example, anxiety disorders to alertness, hypertension to enhanced blood pressure and cardiac output, or, on the other hand, depression and poststress disorders to a lack of ergotropic activity.

Genetic determinants of ergotropic function may contribute to stress vulnerability. Functions of different components of the adrenergic systems have been reported to be altered by gene polymorphisms for adrenergic receptors [2] and tyrosine hydroxylase [3]. However, overseeing data from neuropattern diagnoses of more than one thousand subjects, we feel that pre- and postnatal programming exerts most powerful effects on the noradrenergic system. Patients with a history of pre- and postnatal stress describe themselves as driven, being always in a 'stand-by' mode, ready to go, and seem to be particularly prone to anxiety disorders. However, this awaits confirmation by suited study protocols.

Unfortunately, until now relatively few research studies have focused on these determinants. Epidemiological studies suggest that an unfavorable fetal environment, which results in low birth weight, constitutes an important risk factor for chronic cardiovascular and metabolic diseases in adult life [4]. Lundy et al. [5] found in a prospective study that depressed women had higher cortisol and norepinephrine (NE) and lower dopamine levels during pregnancy and that their newborns also had higher cortisol and NE levels and lower dopamine levels, thus mimicking their mothers' biochemical profile. Stepwise regression analyses showed that the depressed mothers' prenatal NE and dopamine levels significantly predicted the newborns' NE and dopamine levels and behavioral effects as verified by Brazelton scores. Interestingly, Sarkar et al. [6] provided evidence that prenatal stress leading to elevated maternal and/or fetal catecholamine levels may decrease the placental glucocorticoid barrier and, thereby, increase fetal exposure to maternal glucocorticoids. Schneider et al. [7] observed higher MHPG levels in the cerebrospinal fluid (CSF) in the offspring of prenatally stressed rhesus monkeys. In pigs, elevated maternal cortisol during late gestation also produced a significant decrease of plasma CBG, but significantly increased plasma NE [8]. Similar findings were obtained from rats [9]. Such data provide preliminary evidence for prenatal NE programming, and, in consequence, higher responses of target tissues in the offspring of prenatally stressed mothers [10].

Early adverse events in childhood may have similar consequences. Again, while effects on the HPAA have been extensively investigated, there are not too many data on the adrenergic consequences of early adverse experiences. Meaney's group in Montreal used a maternal care model, and found that the density of α_2-autoreceptors in the LC goes up with high maternal care. NE inhibits its own release by presynaptic α_2-receptors and would thus buffer hyperactivity or hyperreactivity of NE. High maternal care was further associated with increased benzodiazepine receptor density in the amygdala and LC, while CRF receptor density in the LC was decreased. These researchers thus assume protective effects of maternal care. Low maternal care, on the other hand, may program a disinhibited NE system and thus promote vulnerability for anxiety and fear in later life. In this animal model, low maternal care was indeed associated with higher fearfulness in animals that had experienced low maternal care [11, 12]. Even for predictable stress, these animals showed higher increases of NE in the PVN.

The literature, however, is still a bit puzzling: effects vary with type, timing and length of intervention, species, gender, genes, rearing conditions, time of outcome measures in development, and, not surprisingly, the central and the peripheral components are sometimes dissociated [13, 14]. However, there seems to be rather consistent evidence on pre-/postnatal programming of enhanced plasma NE levels under both stimulated and unstimulated conditions. Enhanced plasma NE levels have been considered an important risk factor in a recent larger prospective study for metabolic, cardiovascular and reproductive disorders [15].

Finally, it should be noted that sympathetic effects are very complex and regionally regulated in effector organs. Thus, terms like 'sympathetic arousal' are not of high physiological value, but rather provide a preliminary estimate of gross physiological effects. The sympathetic innervation of the immune system, for example, affects the Th1-Th2 balance and has been considered to modulate stress effects on atopic disorders, fibromyalgia, and chronic fatigue syndrome. Although the anatomical and physiological mechanisms behind them are not yet fully understood, pharmacological interventions based on such assumptions are already promising [16]. In other words, the heuristic clinical value is that one can develop an idea how stress compromises the immune system of a patient, and what can be done to prevent or treat these symptoms.

6.2. Ergotropic Endophenotypes

Hyper- and hypoactivity, as well as hyper- and hyporeactivity of the LC and the SNS, may be discriminated to better characterize these interfaces of the crosstalk between the brain and the body. This, however, would imply that altered activity and reactivity of the LC and SNS could be differentiated by suited psychological, biological, and symptom variables.

Hypertension, for example, is strongly promoted by sympathetic outflow [17]. Reasons for enhanced sympathetic outflow are multiple and can be of central or peripheral origin, both being determined by genetic or epigenetic factors. When centrally determined, the noradrenergic stress response can indirectly induce sympathetic activation, mainly via the PVN [1]. Thus, both sympathetic measures and symptoms vary with NE activity. For example, psychological variables (e.g. anger suppression, type A behavior) and biological measures (e.g. catecholamines), both ergotropic in nature, have been linked to hypertension [18]. When determined peripherally, enhanced sympathetic arousal may also evoke psychological changes being perceived as emotions or attributed as anxiety or anger, and thus affect self-reporting of psychological symptoms [19, 20]. A good example for this is pheochromocytoma, a catecholamine-producing tumor, which does not only create the expected bodily symptoms such as sweating, tachycardia and hypertension, but also includes feelings of panic and anxiety [21]. Thus, careful integrative conceptualization and analyses are necessary to differentiate and dissect the specific psychological, biological, and symptomatic measures for each component of the ergotropic systems.

6.2.1. Ergotropic Hyperactivity and Hyperreactivity

Sympathetic activation during psychological stress seems to be primarily mediated by the LC [22]. Under chronic stress, HPAA and sympathetic reactivity dissociate: while HPAA response quickly habituates in most subjects, the sympathetic response remains unchanged [23]. Thus, chronic stress may predominantly affect bodily function via the autonomic pathway. Activation of the LC results in broad effects on many different brain areas, which allow the brain to improve processing of internal and external stimuli. Subjectively, this state is experienced as alertness, arousal and wakefulness, and measures for cognitive performance are improved as soon as there is no overstimulation of the LC [24]. Besides direct mutual inhibition, afferent (autonomic, visceral, somatic) signals and efferent impulses are transmitted to the SNS via the Ncl. paragigantocellularis in the medulla [25].

Noradrenergic hyperactivity refers to an unknown trait that has been attempted to be assessed by psychological and biological measures. It is not yet clear if and how NE hyperactivity can be determined individually. Genetic and epigenetic factors are surely important [2, 13, 26]. Psychological traits are moderately and inconsistently related to blood pressure. In a careful review, Schum et al. [27] addressed the spectrum of methodological difficulties, which may explain inconsistent findings, but his analysis still verified a certain role of trait anger on blood pressure, when assessed by ambulatory monitoring in the natural environment. This may change once we focus on the respective interfaces which participate in the regulation of blood pressure. In a recent review on noradrenergic and serotonergic control mechanisms of blood pressure, Lechin and van der Dijs [28] conclude that essential hypertension depends on the hyperactivity of the neural sympathetic but not the adrenal sympathetic peripheral system. They provide evidence that essential hypertension is predominantly affected by noradrenergic neurons arising from the pontine and medullary regions (A5) and the median raphe nucleus, while the LC acts synergistically with the dorsal raphe nucleus and antagonistically to the median raphe in regulating blood pressure. Obviously, our knowledge is far more precise and predictable as far as these interfaces are concerned. Conceptualizing and assessing the biological, psychological, and symptomatic features of the interfaces may thus help explain more accurately how stress affects essential hypertension.

Similarily, Bunker et al. [29] summarized the results of the Expert Working Group of the National Heart Foundation of Australia, who reviewed the evidence relating coronary heart disease (CHD) to major psychosocial risk factors: 'The expert group concluded that (1) there is strong and consistent evidence of an independent causal association between depression, social isolation and lack of quality social support and the causes and prognosis of CHD, and (2) there is no strong or consistent evidence for a causal association between chronic life events, work-related stressors (job control, demands and strain), type A behavior patterns, hostility, anxiety disorders or panic disorders and CHD.' With respect to stress, the group agreed that acute life stressors can trigger coronary events, but they felt that the term 'stress' is too imprecise to be helpful [29, p. 279].

It seems that psychological traits are not directly relevant for CHD, but they may rather facilitate pathological conditions and impair the ability of an individual to adequately adapt to challenges. For example, CHD and diabetes type 2 often occur as a consequence of obesity and hypertension. Ergotropic determinants are likely to play a crucial role within a complexity of other factors in the development of obesity and elevated blood pressure. So, one may not expect a direct association between such psychological traits and disease outcome. Rather, it seems to be necessary to define such traits with a clear focus on the physiological interface. Thus, in our approach we focussed solely on trait measures of dorsal noradrenergic activity and assessed them by a pattern of psychological (e.g. increased drive, restlessness, nervousness, alertness), biological and symptom variables. Interestingly, these variables seem to vary strongly with pre- and postnatal adversity, and they are also known as risk factors for a subgroup of depression. This needs to be verified in cohort studies.

Evidently, one subgroup seems to develop adiposity under stress due to an enhanced release of neuropeptide Y, a cotransmitter of NE in adipose tissues, which results in a subsequent increase of numbers of adipocytes and fat mass [30]. Indeed, we recently found that healthy students with a history of early adversity already have a greater body mass index and already show evidence for insulin resistance [31, 32]. Activation of the SNS inhibits glucose uptake by peripheral tissues by inhibiting insulin release and inducing insulin resistance and increasing hepatic glucose production. Notably, Kuo et al. [30] found converging effects of glucocorticoids and SNS effects, since stressors also increased the intracellular expression of 11β-hydroxysteroid dehydrogenase-1 in adipocytes, which converts inactive cortisone to active cortisol, thus also promoting fat mass [33, 34]. Osteoporosis, as another disorder associated with depression and the metabolic syndrome, is also affected by increased noradrenergic effects on bones [35].

A regulatory role of the LC has been proposed in anxiety disorders. Psychiatric research has documented that enhanced noradrenergic postsynaptic responsiveness in the neuronal pathway that originates in the LC and ends in the amygdala is a major factor in the pathophysiology of most stress-induced fear-circuitry disorders and especially in post-traumatic stress disorder [36]. In addition, another network of prefrontal brain regions is involved in the cognitive regulation of anxiety and depression

[37, 38]. The interplay between neocortical, allocortical and subcortical structures has been nicely summarized and illustrated by Sullivan et al. [39] and Tanaka et al. [40], suggesting that increased NE release in the hypothalamus, amygdala and LC is the major determinant by which stressful stimuli provoke anxiety or fear. Both overviews impressively demonstrate the extensive evidence for the LC as a major determinant of anxiety disorders, mainly reflecting the stress component.

Acute and chronic exposure to a stressor does not only increase catecholamine turnover and release, but also sensitizes the brain to enhance the reactivity to subsequent stressors [41]. Single administration of the cytokine interleukin-1α (IL-1) or the psychostimulant amphetamine provokes an enhanced and long-lasting hypothalamic-pituitary-adrenal sensitization, which is paralleled by an increase in the electrically evoked release of NE in the PVN [42, 43]. Thus, an ergotropic hyperreactivity may develop as a consequence of acute or chronic stress, which seems to be mainly determined by noradrenergic sensitization. This may particularly promote intrusions in post-traumatic stress disorders (PTSD). In humans, stress-induced NE sensitization is considered to contribute to fear and anxiety disorders, such as PTSD [44]. The LC neurons are probably involved in intrusions in PTSD patients, which may explain the effectiveness of propranolol and prazosin for the secondary prevention and treatment of such symptoms in PTSD [45]. Furthermore, patients with PTSD and panic disturbances react more sensitively to stimulation of the noradrenergic nerves, show higher heart rate reactions and increased levels of catecholamines [46]. Stimulation of the LC creates anxious and fearful behavior, while anxiolytic drugs dampen both the firing rate of the LC and the release of NE. Pre- and postnatal adversity during brain development is likely to facilitate noradrenergic sensitization in later life. Evidence for that has been provided in both animals [11, 12] and humans, and in the latter such determinants seem to constitute later vulnerability for affective disorders [47].

In addition, NE also facilitates conditioning of responses to stressful and fearful stimuli [39, 48, 49], although the precise mechanisms still await to be elucidated [50]. Thus, NE may facilitate both conditioning and sensitization in patients with attention-deficiency hyperactivity disorder (ADHD), post-traumatic stress disorders (PTSD) and panic disorders [46], and some symptoms improve well under treatment with catecholamine antagonists [51, 52].

Activity of the LC is accompanied by activation of the SNS and deactivation of the parasympathetic nervous system. Increases in heart rate, blood pressure, elevated levels of epinephrine and NE, glucose, and suppression of trophotropic functions such as reproduction and digestion have all been observed both after LC stimulation and in states of anxiety and fear. Furthermore, NE hyperactivity and hyperreactivity have both been discussed to be of pathological relevance for several other disorders associated with anxiety, such as hyperventilation, palpitations and pronounced perspiration [39].

Case Report

Our case, a 40-year-old male engineer, suffered from excessive sweating, panic attacks, episodes of tachycardia, prolonged stomach trouble with additional sickness and exaggerated concerns for his health. His family anamnesis revealed hypochondria and mental problems in his mother and his grandmother. His father suffered from restless legs syndrome and died of cancer when our patient was 30 years old, both of his brothers suffered from marked nervousness, increased stress responsivity and pronounced sweating.

During her pregnancy with him, his mother's sister, being pregnant herself, was diagnosed as having leukemia; 10 months after he was born, his aunt died and his mother took care of his 7-month-old cousin. However, she was deeply affected by her sister's death and developed a depression and pronounced hypochondria. When asked about his childhood, he described himself as shy, small compared to children of the same age and socially withdrawn. Very early on, his mother took him to hospitals and administered medicine for the slightest complaints he reported. He states that he has taken over these exaggerated concerns for health from his mother. His complaints, such as sleep disturbances, stomach pain and extreme sweating, were triggered for the first time in a phase of maltreatment by his cotrainees during his apprenticeship. At the same time, he was taking L-thyroxine because of a diagnosed hypothyroidism. His metabolism stabilized after a while, making medication unnecessary. A second-degree struma, however, still persists.

During his training he had an accident, followed by a swelling of his lymph nodes. At the same time, a person he knew died of leukemia. He now developed a strong fear of dying of cancer. Only a tranquillizer was able to calm him down at that time, and he experienced his first panic attack. Before going to psychotherapy in 2001, he suffered daily anxiety attacks with massive sweating, heart palpitations and strong feelings of restlessness, accompanied by irrational thoughts of diseases. After such an attack, he usually suffered stomachache for several days.

Assessment of the HPAA and autonomous nervous system revealed the following biological characteristics: cortisol measured in saliva showed normal values for awakening, but a massive increase of 36 nmol/l within the first 30 min after awakening. In other words, the awakening rise showed an elevated AUC and a high acrophase of 190% increase; however, cortisol levels across the day were normal. After oral application of dexamethasone, the cortisol awakening response was normally suppressed.

Under laboratory stress (Trier Social Stress Test; TSST), the patient showed a marked endocrine stress response. Free cortisol increased by more than 20 nmol/l, thus exaggerating the expected increase of 8 nmol/l. Epinephrine increased from a high baseline level of 141 to 859 pg/ml (expected: 30 pg/ml before and 60 pg/ml during TSST). Thus, a 630% increase of epinephrine was observed in response to psychological stress, while a similar hyperresponsivity of 813% was observed after insulin-induced hypoglycemia. Concurrently, he showed extreme perspiration, even resulting in a wet spot on the floor.

In the neuropattern diagnostic system, the patient qualified for NE hyperactivity and subsequent NE depletion, respectively. In 10 of 11 symptoms, which make up the pattern, his values were above the mean ± SD. A pheochromocytoma, thyroid dysfunction and other possible physical causes of his symptomatology were excluded diagnostically.

We speculate on a genetic and/or acquired (pre-/postnatal) disposition of an increased activity of the LC, which facilitated sensitization of this system by different environmental events (hypochondria of the mother, physical insults, loss of a significant other). Enhanced adrenergic responsivity and, consequently, enhanced perception of bodily events may have facilitated his hypochondria and manifested his complaints.

Mood disorders are not obligatory in stress related bodily disorders. A demonstrative example is male infertility. In a major subgroup of infertile men, depression is actually related to better fertility both in patients and animals. On the contrary, active, dominant and competitive behaviors were found to be associated with low testosterone levels and low sperm count. Activity wheel stress in animals resulted in a strong turnover of NE in many brain areas, accompanied by a vasoconstriction of the blood vessels in the testes. In consequence, luteinizing hormone could not sufficiently stimulate the synthesis and release of testosterone in Leydig cells, finally resulting in a degeneration of spermatids in the testosterone-sensitive stages of maturation. In patients, behavioral therapy turned out to improve coping with stress and significantly increased sperm count and fertility [53]. Thus, an enhanced adrenergic reactivity in both the central and autonomic nervous systems seems to impair fertility. Whether such an effect occurs or not depends primarily on the ergotropic nature of the stress response, and only indirectly on the diverse psychological factors behind.

The LC is further involved in the regulation of pain. Patients with fibromyalgia and chronic fatigue syndrome show an enhanced noradrenergic reactivity to stress [54–56]. In an overview, Pertovaara [57] discriminated (a) peripheral pronociceptive effects, (b) peripheral antinociceptive effects, and (c) pain suppression via NE release from the descending pathways. Sustained pain is considered to induce noradrenergic feedback inhibition of pain. Jorum et al. [58] recently provided evidence that sensitized mechano-insensitive nociceptors can be activated by endogenously released catecholamines and thereby may contribute to sympathetically maintained pain.

Furthermore, patients with fibromyalgia show pronounced sleep disorders and enhanced noradrenergic responsivity to stress [54]. This may possibly be linked to disinhibition of the LC, either by missing inhibitory effects of glucocorticoids (see chapter 5) or the ventrolateral preoptic area of the hypothalamus, which controls the sleep-wake cycle [59]. Such data point to a crucial role of LC hyperactivity in sleep disorders under stress conditions.

Finally, an ergotropic hyperactivity and hyperreactivity can also be determined peripherally. The close bi-directional interaction of the noradrenergic system and the SNS is important, since perception and attribution of ergotropic body signals in the periphery can be interpreted – as stated by the James-Lange theory – as stressful. As mentioned in chapter 3, sympathetic hyperactivity can be caused by a pheochromocytoma, a catecholamine-producing tumor, which thus induces both peripheral symptoms (headaches, sweating, hypertension, palpitations, etc.), and psychological stress (panic and anxiety).

6.2.2. Ergotropic Hypoactivity and Hyporeactivity

NE hypoactivity is characterized by decreased synthesis and release of this neurotransmitter and may be determined by genetic and epigenetic factors at postsynaptic receptor sites. Several neurological and neuropsychiatric diseases have been reported to be associated with NE deficiency, such as depression [60], anorexia nervosa

[61, 62], Parkinson's disease [63], and Alzheimer's disease [64]. It has been discussed that part of the genetic variance can be attributed to a deficit of dopamine-β hydroxylase (DBH), the enzyme which converts dopamine to NE [65]. Under such conditions, the NE deficit can possibly be compensated by adaptation of postsynaptic receptor sites and an enhanced release of co-transmitters [66]. Some evidence suggests that a NE deficiency results in a sensitization of postsynaptic receptor sites [67], resulting in hyperresponsivity of the ergotropic system once strong stressors provoke a high release of NE [61]. Ergotropic responsivity may thus be characterized by the concomitant occurrence of both NE hypoactivity and NE hyperreactivity and may be difficult to discriminate between. However, in terms of etiopathogenesis and treatment this may well be of interest. Notably, it has been suggested that a reduced responsiveness of the LC-NE system could be protective [68].

Under chronic stress, the LC and the synthesis and release of NE are permanently stimulated; if such conditions persist, a depletion of NE storage vesicles will be expected, which cannot be compensated by a sufficient synthesis of this neurotransmitter, allowing the vesicles to refill [69]. Thus, NE depletion is another scenario, which can be observed as a consequence of chronic stress. This status is characterized by an own specific pattern of psychological, biological, and symptomatic characteristics, which are mainly observed under poststress conditions. Symptoms include pronounced fatigue, lack of initiative and motivation and symptoms promoted by low sympathetic but high parasympathetic activity, characteristically occurring not before or during, but particularly after the stress load [70]. Characteristic time periods for complaints are evenings, weekends and vacations.

Mezzacappa et al. [71] observed a vagal rebound during recovery from stress. They discuss this response as a possible predictor of cardiovascular disease. In animals, the occurrence of gastric ulcerations under poststress conditions could be prevented by vagotomy, the NE precursor tyrosine, and yohimbine, an α_2-receptor antagonist which promotes noradrenergic activity [72]. Even in consequence of extreme physical stress, poststress symptoms such as performance incompetence, fatigue, altered mood states, increased rate of infections, and suppressed reproductive functions have been observed. These are associated, among others, with a decrease in β-receptor density and sympathetic activity [73]. In a pilot study of 49 subjects who fulfilled the criteria of burnout, we recently observed that 24 of them qualified for the neuropattern of NE hypoactivity, while the remaining 25 qualified for five different neuropatterns [Horstmann, Kudielka, et al., unpubl.]. Thus, NE depletion is likely to constitute a major determinant of fatigue, burnout, and cognitive impairment.

Reviewing the role of NE depletion, NE turnover, NE receptor density and sensitivity, and effects of antidepressants on the NE system in depression, Nemeroff [74] concluded that NE metabolism may be decreased, increased, or unchanged in patients whose depression is untreated: 'The LC of suicide victims was found to contain signs of increases in tyrosine hydroxylase activity and an increased density of α_2-adrenergic autoreceptors, an observation also noted in rats subjected to either chronic stimulation of the LC or NE depletion. This may indicate that excessive stimulation of the LC leads to depletion of endogenous NE and a corresponding increase in the levels of synthetic enzymes and upregulation of autoreceptors.' Interestingly, most antidepressants need an intact noradrenergic system to exert their effects [75]. The therapeutic effects of psychotherapy and behavioral activity (active coping, jogging, etc.) may potentially be transmitted by this route to the LC [76] although different receptor systems seem to be involved [77].

Again, peripheral events may also contribute to symptomatology. As mentioned in chapter 3, patients with diabetes and uremia often develop a peripheral sympathetic neuropathy and heart failure. These and other diseases of the SNS may result in sympathetic dysfunction. In some patients, low catecholamine levels are associated with enhanced stress responsivity, suggesting a compensatory upregulation of postsynaptic receptors, and one may expect that both physical and psychological stresses provoke strong sympathetic neuronal responses [78]. Comparably, lower plasma NE levels have been observed in patients with supine hypertension [79].

In sum, to fully understand the ergotropic stress response, it may occasionally be relevant to include assessments of sympathetic reactivity to stress. Hyperresponsive patients may have either a high or a low basal sympathetic tone. To obtain a useful diagnosis, it seems necessary to include a careful assessment of peripheral sympathetic arousal. Both the dorsal noradrenergic bundles originating in the LC and those in the SNS seem to act synergistically in terms of ergotropic stress response.

6.3. Summary

The dorsal noradrenergic system and the SNS seem to synchronize the activity and reactivity of the organism and constitute the major systems involved in the ergotropic stress response. The sensitivity of these systems is affected by numerous biological and environmental factors. Symptoms of physical and mental stress vary with the activity and reactivity of these systems. Assessing the status of both the LC and the SNS is mandatory in the diagnosis of stress-related disorders.

References

1 Benarroch EE: Paraventricular nucleus, stress response, and cardiovascular disease. Clin Auton Res 2005;15:254–263.

2 Kirstein SL, Insel PA: Autonomic nervous system pharmacogenomics: a progress report. Pharmacol Rev 2004;56:31–52.

3 Zhang L, Rao F, Wessel J, Kennedy BP, Rana BK, Taupenot L, Lillie EO, Cockburn M, Schork NJ, Ziegler MG, O'Connor DT: Functional allelic heterogeneity and pleiotropy of a repeat polymorphism in tyrosine hydroxylase: prediction of catecholamines and response to stress in twins. Physiol Genomics 2004;19:277–291.

4 Barker DJP: Fetal Origins of Cardiovascular and Lung Disease. New York, Marcel Dekker, 2001.

5 Lundy BL, Jones NA, Field T, Nearing G, Davalos M, Pietro PA, Schanberg S, Kuhn C: Prenatal depression effects on neonates. Infant Behav Dev 1999;22:119–129.

6 Sarkar S, Tsai SW, Nguyen TT, Plevyak M, Padbury JF, Rubin LP: Inhibition of placental 11beta-hydroxysteroid dehydrogenase type 2 by catecholamines via alpha-adrenergic signaling. Am J Physiol 2001;281:R1966–R1974.
7 Schneider ML, Clarke AS, Kraemer GW, Roughton EC, Lubach GR, Rimm-Kaufman S, Schmidt D, Ebert M: Prenatal stress alters brain biogenic amine levels in primates. Dev Psychopathol 1998;10:427–440.
8 Kanitz E, Otten W, Tuchscherer M: Changes in endocrine and neurochemical profiles in neonatal pigs prenatally exposed to increased maternal cortisol. J Endocrinol 2006;191:207–220.
9 Lesage J, Dufourny L, Laborie C, Bernet F, Blondeau B, Avril I, Breant B, Dupouy JP: Perinatal malnutrition programs sympathoadrenal and hypothalamic-pituitary-adrenal axis responsiveness to restraint stress in adult male rats. J Neuroendocrinol 2002; 14:135–143.
10 Deruelle P, Houfflin-Debarge V, Magnenant E, Jaillard S, Riou Y, Puech F, Storme L: Effects of antenatal glucocorticoids on pulmonary vascular reactivity in the ovine fetus. Am J Obstet Gynecol 2003;189:208–215.
11 Caldji C, Tannenbaum B, Sharma S, Francis D, Plotsky PM, Meaney MJ: Maternal care during infancy regulates the development of neural systems mediating the expression of fearfulness in the rat. Proc Natl Acad Sci USA 1998;95:5335–5340.
12 Liu D, Caldji C, Sharma S, Plotsky PM, Meaney MJ: Influence of neonatal rearing conditions on stress-induced adrenocorticotropin responses and norepinepherine release in the hypothalamic paraventricular nucleus. J Neuroendocrinol 2000;12:5–12.
13 Holmes A, le Guisquet AM, Vogel E, Millstein RA, Leman S, Belzung C: Early life genetic, epigenetic and environmental factors shaping emotionality in rodents. Neurosci Biobehav Rev 2005;29:1335–1346.
14 Matthews K, Dalley JW, Matthews C, Tsai TH, Robbins TW: Periodic maternal separation of neonatal rats produces region- and gender-specific effects on biogenic amine content in postmortem adult brain. Synapse 2001;40:1–10.
15 Gruenewald TL, Seeman TE, Ryff CD, Karlamangla AS, Singer BH: Combinations of biomarkers predictive of later life mortality. Proc Natl Acad Sci USA 2006;103:14158–14163.
16 Elenkov IJ, Wilder RL, Chrousos GP, Vizi ES: The sympathetic nerve – an integrative interface between two supersystems: the brain and the immune system. Pharmacol Rev 2000;52:595–638.
17 Guyenet PG: The sympathetic control of blood pressure. Nat Rev 2006;7:335–346.
18 Vogele C, Jarvis A, Cheeseman K: Anger suppression, reactivity, and hypertension risk: gender makes a difference. Ann Behav Med 1997;19:61–69.
19 Craig AD: Human feelings: Why are some more aware than others? Trends Cogn Sci 2004;8:239–241.
20 Schachter S, Singer JE: Cognitive, social, and physiological determinants of emotional state. Psychol Rev 1962;69:379–399.
21 Zelinka T, Eisenhofer G, Pacak K: Pheochromocytoma as a catecholamine producing tumor: implications for clinical practice. Stress 2007;10:195–203.
22 Charmandari E, Tsigos C, Chrousos G: Endocrinology of the stress response. Ann Rev Physiol 2005;67:259–284.
23 Schommer NC, Hellhammer DH, Kirschbaum C: Dissociation between reactivity of the hypothalamus-pituitary-adrenal axis and the sympathetic-adrenal-medullary system to repeated psychosocial stress. Psychosom Med 2003;65:450–460.
24 Foote S, Aston-Jones G: Pharmacology and physiology of central noradrenergic systems; in Bloom F, DK (eds): Psychopharmacology: The Fourth Generation of Progress. New York, Raven Press, 1995, pp 335–345.
25 Valentino RJ, Aston-Jones GS: Physiological and anatomical determinants of locus coeruleus discharge; in Bloom F, Kupfer D (eds): Psychopharmacology: The Fourth Generation of Progress. New York, Raven Press, 1995, pp 373–385.
26 Jabbi M, Kema IP, van der Pompe G, te Meerman GJ, Ormel J, den Boer JA: Catechol-o-methyltransferase polymorphism and susceptibility to major depressive disorder modulates psychological stress response. Psychiatr Genet 2007;17:183–193.
27 Schum JL, Jorgensen RS, Verhaeghen P, Sauro M, Thibodeau R: Trait anger, anger expression, and ambulatory blood pressure: a meta-analytic review. J Behav Med 2003;26:395–415.
28 Lechin F, van der Dijs B: Central nervous system circuitry and peripheral neural sympathetic activity responsible for essential hypertension. Curr Neurovasc Res 2006;3:307–325.
29 Bunker SJ, Colquhoun DM, Esler MD, Hickie IB, Hunt D, Jelinek VM, Oldenburg BF, Peach HG, Ruth D, Tennant CC, Tonkin AM: 'Stress' and coronary heart disease: psychosocial risk factors. Med J Austr 2003;178:272–276.
30 Kuo LE, Kitlinska JB, Tilan JU, Li L, Baker SB, Johnson MD, Lee EW, Burnett MS, Fricke ST, Kvetnansky R, Herzog H, Zukowska Z: Neuropeptide Y acts directly in the periphery on fat tissue and mediates stress-induced obesity and metabolic syndrome. Nat Med 2007;13:803–811.

31 Entringer S: Exposure to Prenatal Psychosocial Stress: Implications for Long-Term Disease Susceptibility. Göttingen, Cuvillier, 2007.
32 Entringer S, Wüst S, Kumsta R, Layer I, Nelson EL, Wadhwa PD: Prenatal stress is associated with insulin resistance in young adults. Am J Gynecol Obstetr; submitted.
33 Hochberg Z, Friedberg M, Yaniv L, Bader T, Tiosano D: Hypothalamic regulation of adiposity: the role of 11beta-hydroxysteroid dehydrogenase type 1. Hormon Stoffwechselforsch 2004;36:365–369.
34 Levitt NS, Lambert EV, Woods D, Hales CN, Andrew R, Seckl JR: Impaired glucose tolerance and elevated blood pressure in low birth weight, nonobese, young South African adults: early programming of the cortisol axis. J Clin Endocrinol Metab 2000;85:4611–4618.
35 Yirmiya R, Goshen I, Bajayo A, Kreisel T, Feldman S, Tam J, Trembovler V, Csernus V, Shohami E, Bab I: Depression induces bone loss through stimulation of the sympathetic nervous system. Proc Natl Acad Sci USA 2006;103:16876–16881.
36 Kimble M, Kaufman M: Clinical correlates of neurological change in posttraumatic stress disorder: an overview of critical systems. Psychiatr Clin N Am 2004;27:49–65, viii.
37 Davidson RJ: Anxiety and affective style: role of prefrontal cortex and amygdala. Biol Psychiatry 2002;51:68–80.
38 Mayberg H: Depression. II. Localization of pathophysiology. Am J Psychiatry 2002;159:1979.
39 Sullivan RM, Gratton A: Lateralized effects of medial prefrontal cortex lesions on neuroendocrine and autonomic stress responses in rats. J Neurosci 1999;19:2834–2840.
40 Tanaka M, Yoshida M, Emoto H, Ishii H: Noradrenaline systems in the hypothalamus, amygdala and locus coeruleus are involved in the provocation of anxiety: basic studies. Eur J Pharmacol 2000;405:397–406.
41 Gresch PJ, Sved AF, Zigmond MJ, Finlay JM: Stress-induced sensitization of dopamine and norepinephrine efflux in medial prefrontal cortex of the rat. J Neurochem 1994;63:575–583.
42 Jansen AS, Schmidt ED, Voorn P, Tilders FJ: Substance induced plasticity in noradrenergic innervation of the paraventricular hypothalamic nucleus. Eur J Neurosci 2003;17:298–306.
43 Schmidt ED, Schoffelmeer AN, De Vries TJ, Wardeh G, Dogterom G, Bol JG, Binnekade R, Tilders FJ: A single administration of interleukin-1 or amphetamine induces long-lasting increases in evoked noradrenaline release in the hypothalamus and sensitization of ACTH and corticosterone responses in rats. Eur J Neurosci 2001;13:1923–1930.
44 Bremner JD, Krystal JH, Southwick SM, Charney DS: Noradrenergic mechanisms in stress and anxiety: I. Preclinical studies. Synapse 1996;23:28–38.
45 Debiec J, Altemus M: Toward a new treatment for traumatic memories. Cerebrum 2006:2–11.
46 Charney SD, Bremner JD, Redmond DE Jr: Noradrenergic neural substrates for anxiety and fear: clinical associations based on preclinical research; in Bloom EF, Kupfer JD (eds): Psychopharmacology: The Fourth Generation of Progress. New York, Raven Press, 1995, pp 387–395.
47 Heim C, Nemeroff CB: The role of childhood trauma in the neurobiology of mood and anxiety disorders: preclinical and clinical studies. Biol Psychiatry 2001;49:1023–1039.
48 Feenstra MG: Dopamine and noradrenaline release in the prefrontal cortex in relation to unconditioned and conditioned stress and reward. Prog Brain Res 2000;126:133–163.
49 Ninan PT: The functional anatomy, neurochemistry, and pharmacology of anxiety. J Clin Psychiatry 1999;60(suppl 22):12–17.
50 Harley CW: Norepinephrine and dopamine as learning signals. Neural Plasticity 2004;11:191–204.
51 Raskind MA, Peskind ER, Hoff DJ, Hart KL, Holmes HA, Warren D, Shofer J, O'Connell J, Taylor F, Gross C, Rohde K, McFall ME: A parallel group placebo controlled study of prazosin for trauma nightmares and sleep disturbance in combat veterans with post-traumatic stress disorder. Biol Psychiatry 2007;61:928–934.
52 Strawn JR, Geracioti TD Jr: Noradrenergic dysfunction and the psychopharmacology of posttraumatic stress disorder. Depress Anxiety 2007;Mar12 [Epub ahead of print].
53 Hellhammer DH, Gutberlet I: Male infertility: Preliminary evidence for two neuroendocrine mediators of stress on gonadal function; in Ferrendelli JA, Collins RC, Johnson EA (eds): Neurobiology of Amino Acids, Peptides and Trophic Factors. Boston, Kluwer Academic Publishers, 1988, pp 227–230.
54 Hesse-Husain J: Fibromyalgia: a psychoneuroimmunological perspective. Trier, University of Trier, 2007.
55 Torpy DJ, Papanicolaou DA, Lotsikas AJ, Wilder RL, Chrousos GP, Pillemer SR: Responses of the sympathetic nervous system and the hypothalamic-pituitary-adrenal axis to interleukin-6: a pilot study in fibromyalgia. Arthritis Rheum 2000;43:872–880.
56 Tsigos C, Chrousos GP: Hypothalamic-pituitary-adrenal axis, neuroendocrine factors and stress. J Psychosom Res 2002;53:865–871.
57 Pertovaara A: Noradrenergic pain modulation. Prog Neurobiol 2006;80:53–83.

we definitively have to acknowledge the (temporary) usefulness of concepts, preferably those which implicate system function.

In biological psychiatry, most concepts refer to symptoms and diseases, and only very few to function. With respect to stress-related disorders, McEwen [6] conceptualized vulnerability factors as allostasis and allostatic load, while Charney [7] emphasized the role of protective factors in resilience to stress. Both concepts were highly important and stimulating for translational stress research. They both dissected and integrated the available knowledge on different (neuro-)endocrine modulators and brain function, thus facilitating translational approaches. Our own concept on glandotropy, ergotropy, and trophotropy (chapter 3) primarily refers to physiological systems and principles, and only secondarily to the neuromodulators involved (biogenic amines, peptides, hormones). Given the diversity of brain functions during development, it is unlikely that only one or two trophotropic subsystems exist, as in the ANS. Rather, several subsystems seem to buffer stress, using different neurotransmitters such as indolamines (e.g. serotonin, melatonin), amino acids (e.g. GABA) and proteins (e.g. brain-derived neurotrophic factor), while their overall function is only partly understood.

In this chapter, we mainly focus on the DR and the parasympathetic nervous system from a trophotropic perspective. We hope to better understand the nature of these systems in stress pathology. As addressed in chapter 3, we assume (a) stress vulnerability, once trophotropic functions are compromised, and (b) stress protection, which, however, may even become pathological under extreme stress conditions.

7.1. Determinants of Trophotropy

As described in chapter 3, the DR is the major serotonergic nucleus involved in the regulation of psychological stress. Serotonin release is under the tonic inhibitory control of 5-HT_{1A} receptors, which seems to represent trophotropic serotonergic functions. The highest density of (postsynaptic) 5-HT_{1A} receptors is in the hippocampus, while the presynaptic somatodendritic 5-HT_{1A} autoreceptors are primarily located in the raphe nuclei. The function of 5-HT_{1A} autoreceptors is to dampen neuronal firing, 5-HT synthesis, and release of serotonergic neurons. Charney [7] mentioned a specific role of the 5-HT_{1A} receptors in resilience, mediating anxiolytic effects and recovery. With respect to a possible antagonism between trophotropic and ergotropic functions, such effects of 5-HT_{1A} receptors may relate to the amygdala and the hippocampus, and, in addition, to serotonergic projections from the DR to the locus coeruleus [8, 9]. Stress-elevated glucocorticoids reduce the density of 5-HT_{1A} receptors [10], thus possibly attenuating trophotropic serotonergic effects. The antagonistic effects on the locus coeruleus, the amygdala and the hippocampus should phenotypically result in reduced arousal, anxiety, fear and aggression [9, 11].

Hyper- and hyposerotonergic states or traits both seem to be stable and may affect stress vulnerability and stress protection. The effects of stressors vary with such trait factors, which could affect one or more discrete components of the serotonergic system. The DR is activated by a variety of metabolic, psychological, and physical stressors. These effects are rather related to the arousal-evoking quality of the stressor, but vary with the severity and predictability of the stressor, as well as with genetic and developmental determinants [12].

As shown in chapter 3, most relevant trait components are genetic and epigenetic factors. Polymorphisms of the serotonin transporter (5-HTT), for example, make individuals more prone to stress [13] and determine the effects of selective serotonin reuptake inhibitors (SSRI) [14].

The genetic locus causing serotonin uptake involves a polymorphic region (5-HTTLPR) in the promoter region of the gene for the 5-HTT. This gene itself exists as several alleles, the short 'S' allele and the long 'L' allele. The S variant is associated with less, and the L variant with more expression of the transporter protein. Due to an enhanced reuptake, LL carriers may thus show less serotonin availability in the synaptic cleft and, in addition, an enhanced metabolism of serotonin to 5-HIAA. The opposite should be true for SS subjects. Since there is evidence for that, one would further expect that serotonergic transmission is more efficient in SS carriers. However, just the opposite has been observed: SS carriers express more anxiety-related personality traits, show fewer problem-solving strategies for and an enhanced vulnerability to stress and depression, and respond more sensitively to fearful stimuli, but are less sensitive to SSRI [15–18]. A reason for these paradoxical findings is that the serotonergic system counter-regulates the respective 5-HTT availability early by a number of other factors such as expression of pre- and postsynaptic receptors and other proteins in the presynaptic terminals and postsynaptic neurons on neuronal networks [19–23]. It seems that environmental, psychological, or pharmacological manipulations of serotonergic neurotransmission affect this interplay and explain (the time course of) different effects in SS, SL or LL carriers. However, the mechanisms behind them still remain to be fully elucidated.

Prenatal factors such as SSRI treatment of the pregnant mother, depression and stress have been discussed to affect the maturation and function of serotonergic systems in the brain and create a risk for behavioral disturbances and disorders (e.g. autism) in the offspring [24, 25]. Early adverse experiences result under stress conditions in adulthood in an enhanced response of serotonergic neurons, projecting from the DR to the central and autonomic control systems [26]. Field et al. [27, 28] provided evidence on the prenatal programming of low vagal tone in offspring of mothers who scored high on measures of anxiety, depression, and anger in the second trimester of pregnancy. Interestingly, these mothers had also a low vagal tone, possibly suggesting an ergotropic dominance in these subjects, which may be genetically or epigenetically determined.

Gene × environment interactions for stress-related serotonergic functions have been reported for depression [29, 30], cardiovascular diseases [31], aggression [32] lupus nephritis [33], and post-traumatic stress disorder [34]. Although consistently, most studies only explain moderate amounts of variance, since state factors such as the predictability or type and duration of stressors finally affect the outcome of the pathology [35].

In addition, the endocrine milieu impacts on serotonergic- and parasympathetic-modulated functions. Serotonergic states are clearly affected by estrogens and progestins at various cellular levels, which may explain part of the genetic variance of the trophotropic stress response. Gonadal hormones affect serotonergic-modulated functions such as arousal, mood, cognition, pain and hormone secretion [36, 37] and baroreceptor reflexes, especially cardiac outflow [38]. Thyroid hormones also increase serotonergic function, particularly those regulated by the 5-HT_{1A} autoreceptor in the DR and the 5-HT_2 receptor. Thyroid hormones have thus been applied as co-therapeutics in antidepressant treatments [39].

7.2. Trophotropic Endophenotypes

If one wants to assess central and peripheral trophotropic endophenotypes, one should ask how both subtypes are represented and how they interact, and, further, how they participate in stress vulnerability and stress protection. Clearly, the serotonergic system is not a simple trophotropic system in the brain, which behaves agonistically to the parasympathetic system, and which is counter-regulated by ergotropic systems. This counter-regulation is complementary in nature rather than being antagonistic. By balancing ergotropic and trophotropic adaptation to stress, the autonomic nervous system perfectly regulates organ functions during and after stress. In the brain, noradrenergic functions resemble peripheral sympathetic functions, and both ergotropic systems together perfectly interact and adapt to fight, flight or other ergotropic demands. The intriguing neuroanatomical, physiological, and developmental parallels of both monoaminergic systems, however, and the fact that a serotonin deficiency represents the most prominent deficit in trophotropic functions (see 7.2.2.), challenge us to explore a possible underlying 'wisdom of the body'.

7.2.1. Serotonergic Hyperactivity and Hyperreactivity

Hyperactivity of serotonergic and parasympathetic tone in stress-related disorders has rarely been described, since enhanced serotonin function is usually not considered a vulnerability factor, but, rather, 'a stabilizer of neural as well as social networks' [40, p. 3]. However, one may expect higher serotonin turnover in subjects that are genetically predisposed to enhanced serotonin reuptake. The expression of 5-HTT is programmed during fetal life [41] and serotonin reuptake is modulated by a polymorphic repetitive element, the 5-HTT gene-linked polymorphic region, 5-HTTLPR. Carriers of the l-allele are supposed to express more 5-HTT. An enhanced reuptake is probably associated with an enhanced metabolism of serotonin to 5-HIAA. In addition, 5-HT_{1A} autoreceptors may adapt, finally resulting in a normal-to-enhanced serotonergic tone [42]. Thus, under unstimulated conditions these subjects may express a trophotropic phenotype, while showing a deficit to terminate a cardiovascular stress response via 5-HT_{1A} autoreceptors. Indeed, l-allele carriers show higher 5-HIAA levels in the cerebrospinal fluid (CSF), score low on measures of hostility, impulsivity, anger, depression and anxiety, but show an enhanced blood pressure response to stress.

A typical trophotropic stress response is that what has been earlier conceptualized as 'learned helplessness' [43–45] and 'conservation withdrawal behavior' [46]. Both models have a two-phase model in common: after unsuccessful attempts to cope with a stressor, animals and people emit a passive coping response. This passive response has either been interpreted as helplessness or as withdrawal from wasting energy with unsuccessful activities and, instead, conserving energy by behaving inactively. Both concepts are still prominent models of reactive or psychogenic depression. Rats, when exposed to uncontrollable stress, first try all kind of coping attempts and these activities are accompanied by enhanced noradrenergic activities. Under repeated stress, however, active coping attempts continuously decrease, while freezing behavior and serotonergic turnover increases [47]. Observations in primates show a positive correlation between freezing and activity of the DR [48]. Maier and Watkins [35] recently summarized evidence that these effects are mediated by the DR, emphasizing a role of CRF as a sensitizer of serotonergic neurons in the DR. Comparable to sensitization of the noradrenergic response to stress, sensitization of the serotonin response was reported early. Immobilization after chronic restraint decreased 5-HT, increased 5-HIAA, and decreased NA in most brain regions, and seems to sensitize both monoaminergic systems to an additional acute stress [49]. Jezova and Duncko [50] treated healthy volunteers for a week with citalopram and observed an enhanced response of ACTH, growth hormone, prolactin, and systolic blood pressure to insulin-induced hypoglycemia, suggesting a serotonergic sensitization of the stress response.

Case Report

The patient, a 52-year-old patient, suffers from ulcerative colitis. He is divorced and has lost contact with his two children. He first developed ulcerative colitis under marital distress. Due to his disease, he was unable to work and had to retire some years ago. No evidence for pre- or postnatal adversity could be detected. His grandmother, his mother, and his brother all suffered from depression. However, he had a very dominant father who insisted that he showed his best performance in school and always behaved well at home. The patient reports loss of control as a child and describes himself as being shy and anxious during childhood. In school, he had a permanent fear of failure and already realized an association between stressful demands and physical symptoms, e.g. sweating and stomach problems.

In the Neuropattern diagnosis, the patient scored high on psychological measures of passive coping, learned helplessness, loss of appetite under stress, and tiredness. Furthermore, he showed evidence for a sympathetic-parasympathetic imbalance, as evident from an orthostatic syndrome. His cortisol levels were in the normal range, although the awakening response was slightly blunted. No abnormalities after dexamethasone were detected. He further expressed several symptoms, such as gut disorders under stressful conditions, exhaustion, and pain. All in all, he qualified for one pattern only, namely 'serotonin hyperreactivity', with some additional evidence for 'parasympathetic hyperreactivity'.

One may assume that the patient had a history of 'learned helplessness', mainly as a consequence of his father's dominant behavior. A permanent loss of control, perhaps associated with a familiar disposition for depression, let him become anxious and shy in childhood. Later in life, this passive coping behavior has probably generalized to other social situations, restraining him to adequately cope and communicate with his wife and children. He avoided conflicts by withdrawing from social interactions, going into his room and fading out the adverse events. Then, under marital distress, he was only able to emit a trophotropic stress response, probably associated with enhanced serotonergic and parasympathetic activity. During psychotherapy, the patient provided evidence of a close temporal relationship between a passive coping response to stress and diarrhea, suggesting an immediate facilitating effect of a passive coping response on gut pathology.

Opposite to the fight/flight response, Engel and Schmale [46] considered conservation-withdrawal behavior as a risk factor for several somatic disorders, particularly parasympathetic-modulated symptoms such as bradycardia, hypotonia, gastrointestinal complaints, and asthma. In animal experiments, the conservation-withdrawal response is associated with enhanced serotonin levels and gastric ulceration [47, 51]. Social stress has been shown to be associated with serotonergic activity in the DR. Animals with a history of maternal separation showed a passive submissive and less proactive coping response, suggesting a role of early adverse experience in withdrawal behavior [26]. Clinical observations provided evidence that this coping response to stress facilitates diarrhea and pain in patients suffering from colitis ulcerosa [52]. Interestingly, 'learned helplessness' can easily generalize to others but the original stressors [43]. Apart from sensitization, learning may thus be another mechanism that contributes to a trait component of this phenotype.

Notably, peripheral serotonin is involved in such diverse functions as regulation of enteric reflexes, modulation of platelet shape change and blood aggregation, modulation of vascular smooth muscle contraction, initiation of activity in primary afferent nociceptors, and regulation of lymphocyte cytotoxicity and phagocytosis [53, 54]. Thus, gene polymorphisms related to alterations of serotonin function may not only affect stress responsitivity of the brain, but also the vulnerability of bodily functions.

7.2.2. Parasympathetic Hyperactivity and Hyperreactivity

As shown in chapter 3, the response of the parasympathetic nervous system to stress is indirect, and thus needs to be assessed separately. In a recent review in 2007, Vaddadi's group [55] discriminated five forms of postural syncope, which are all related to high parasympathetic tone:

(1) The vasovagal syncope ('blackout') is characterized by sudden hypotension and bradycardia, and can occur after prolonged standing or sitting in response to venepuncture, pain or emotion. Symptoms consistent with vasovagal syncope and most predictive of the diagnosis include visual blurring, sweating, nausea, warmth, lightheadedness and fatigue.

(2) Postural tachycardia syndrome most commonly affects young women and is characterized by fatigue, palpitations, exercise intolerance, light-headedness, visual blurring, chest pain, inability to concentrate and episodic syncope or presyncope. Anxiety and depression are frequent comorbidities.

(3) Chronic autonomic failure is a rare condition which causes orthostatic intolerance. It is associated with degeneration of sympathetic nerves or the central nervous system, diabetic autonomic neuropathy and Parkinsonism with autonomic failure. In the elderly, related symptoms such as fatigue, orthostatic intolerance, erectile dysfunction, urinary retention, loss of sweating, pain in the neck and shoulders, abdominal discomfort and diarrhea may be misattributed as 'psychosomatic symptoms.'

(4) Persistently low supine systolic blood pressure is a recently recognized condition, characterized by low resting sympathetic activity, low blood pressure and proneness to vasovagal events: 'Systolic blood pressure can easily fall to 80 mm Hg as a result of minimal dehydration or drinking a small amount of alcohol. In clinical practice we find this to be a common cause of syncope – patients frequently complain of ongoing fatigue and may also have a prominent tachycardia during orthostasis'.

(5) Initial orthostatic hypotension is mostly observed in young adults a few seconds after standing up.

Apart from direct effects on innervated organ systems, indirect effects on immune functions have also been discussed. Recent evidence suggests that the vagus exerts immunosuppressive effects [55]. Hamer and Steptoe [56] recently showed a smaller inflammatory cytokine response to mental stress, associated with low exercise heart rate, suggesting positive effects of physiological fitness by enhanced vagal tone. In summary, parasympathetic hyperactivity and hyperreactivity may facilitate the trophotropic but buffer the ergotropic stress response. In addition, high vagal tone may alter visceral perception of the stress response. Dorr et al. [57] showed that vagal stimulation increases the firing rate of serotonergic neurons in the brain after 2 weeks. Clinically, vagus nerve stimulation has been shown to be useful in the treatment of severe depression [58]. These and other studies suggest that vagal activity affects emotion as well as cognition.

7.2.3. Serotonergic Hypoactivity and Hyporeactivity

As described in chapter 3, serotonin hypoactivity may become highly relevant for a maladaptive stress response, and experiments using tryptophan depletion have shown that a serotonin deficiency is associated with profound changes in mood and bodily function. The frequent use of SSRIs in stress-related disorders may underline the presence of symptoms of serotonin deficiency in the population. Thus, a serotonin hypoactivity or hyporeactivity can be expected to profoundly contribute to stress pathology. We will here address some of these disorders:

Depression: Mild forms of depression respond well to SSRI, suggesting early that a deficit of serotonin is a major cause of depression. Further evidence came from studies showing low 5-HT and metabolites in postmortem tissues and cerebrospinal fluid, selective depletion studies of 5-HT in depressed patients, and neuroimaging studies. It seems that the deficit of 5-HT in depression is caused by an enhanced reuptake and metabolism of 5-HT. In consequence, less serotonin is available at the synaptic cleft. This results in an upregulation of pre- and postsynaptic receptors. SSRI, which inhibit the reuptake of 5-HT, result in a higher availability of serotonin in the synaptic cleft, and, in consequence, a normalization of pre- and postsynaptic serotonin receptors, explaining the delayed antidepressant effects of SSRI [59–61]. Stressful experiences enhance the risk of major depression, dysregulate the endocrine, autonomic, and immunological stress response, and seem to be the major determinants of risks for physical comorbidity, especially when the stress load occurred during pre- and postnatal development [62–64]. The risk for stress effects on depression is particularly pronounced in carriers of the s-variant of the 5-HTTLPR, who express smaller amounts of 5-HTT [13, 30].

Anxiety disorders: Several studies provided evidence for a partial involvement of serotonin in anxiety disorders. However, study results are still controversial [65]. Neumeister et al. [66] reported reduced 5-HT_{1A} receptor binding in panic disorders, and these receptors have been shown to mediate anxiolytic effects [67]. Furthermore, SSRIs have been approved for treatment of all anxiety disorders and they seem to be also efficient in patients without comorbid depression [68]. Hypoactivity of 5-HT in anxiety disorders may rather facilitate than cause anxiety disorders. Carriers of the short variant of the 5-HTTLPR respond more anxiously and emotionally to stressors [69].

Obsessive-compulsive disorders (OCD): About half of the patients with OCD present comorbidity with major depression, and about 30–40% respond well to SSRIs [70]. However, the role of serotonin does not seem to be causal, but is probably limited to inhibit the orbitofrontal-subcortical circuits involved in OCD [71, 72].

Aggression and impulsivity: Aggression and impulsivity are regulated by numerous neuroendocrine mechanisms. In a recent review, Craig [32] summarized the present knowledge on the link between aggression and stress, and emphasized the role of serotonin. The 'low serotonin syndrome' refers to observations on low 5-HT levels (as evident from CSF, postmortem tissue, and neuroimaging studies) of individuals manifesting persistent impulsive, externally directed aggression, violent suicidal behavior and violent impulsivity, suggesting that lower serotonergic activity is related to aggression. Polymorphisms of the serotonin metabolizing enzyme A (MAO_A) and 5-HTT genes, which result in diminished uptake and metabolism of 5-HT, have been associated with aggression. Further evidence came from studies showing a functional interaction between stress, MAO_A, 5-HTT, and aggression. In rodents, both 5-HTT and MAO_A are activated under social stress, facilitating the uptake and degradation of 5-HT. Craig [32, p. 230] considers this 'a compensatory response to activation of the serotonergic system by the social stress.' This compensatory response may be diminished in carriers of such polymorphisms and make them possibly more vulnerable to an impulsive and aggressive stress response. Early adversity and chronic stress associated with hypocortisolism create another scenario which facilitates aggressive behavior [73] in a predictable time course [74]. Thus, one may expect a beneficial effect of SSRI in aggression. In a recent review, Chamberlain and Sahakian [75], however, do not see enough evidence that pharmacological manipulations of the serotonergic system have detectable behavioral effects on response inhibition.

Cognitive disorders: Rapid tryptophan depletion results in impairment of delayed recall, recognition, and other cognitive performances associated with serotonergic prefrontal functions, particularly with those involving emotional processing [76]. However, contradictory results have also been reported [77], favoring an inverted-U model of cognitive performance [78]. Recently remitted depressed patients treated with SSRI show a remission of depression after tryptophan depletion, with cognitive symptoms such as decreased concentration, loss of energy, ruminative thinking, and sense of worthlessness [79].

Premenstrual syndrome (PMS) and premenstrual dysphoric disorder (PMDD): PMS and PMDD are distinguished by the severity of (mood) symptoms and psychosocial functioning, and both are associated with serotonin hypoactivity, which is probably represented by a decrease of 5-HT_{2C} receptors during the (luteal) premenstrual phase. The surge in female sex steroids impairs 5-HT_{2C} receptor function, and, in consequence, carbohydrate craving, fatigue, and hypersomnia [80]. According to Steiner et al. [81], application of SSRIs is the treatment of choice in these disorders and can prevent menstrual exacerbation of a mood or anxiety disorder.

Eating disorders: Serotonin is one of multiple mediators of eating behavior. In a recent review, Halford et al. [82] summarized the current knowledge on the role of serotonin in eating behavior and on the effects of serotonergic drugs on appetite expression and in the treatment of obesity. The authors show evidence that the hypothalamic serotonin satiety system inhibits feeding behavior within a close network of other modulators such as neuropeptide Y and orexin. 5-HT blocks hunger signals and the hypophagic effect of serotonergic drugs seems to involve the melanocortin system: 'Therefore, as an episodic satiety transmitter, serotonin (like the tonic adiposity signal leptin) influences feeding behavior via both stimulatory and inhibitory effects on several regulatory neuropeptide systems in the hypothalamus.' The 5-HT_{1B}, the 5-HT_{2C} and, possibly, the 5-HT_6 receptors are the key mediators of serotonergic effects. Agonists of the 5-HT_{2C} receptor (chlorphenylpiperazine; mCPP), 5-HTP, and some SSRIs attenuate body weight in rodents, and reduce appetite and caloric intake in humans. In sum, serotonin hypoactivity and the related mood disturbances mentioned here are likely to be associated with enhanced food intake and weight gain. Food intake, preferentially of carbohydrates, may allow individuals to regulate their own serotonin turnover in the brain. Carbohydrates result in an increase of insulin and, consequently, in an enhanced transport of tryptophan into the brain, which is directly converted to serotonin. These mechanisms may be of particular importance under stressful conditions, given the positive effects of serotonin on mood and relaxation [83].

Metabolic syndrome: According to Williams [84, p. 2213], 5-HT hypoactivity 'is a neurobiological substrate that could account for the clustering of psychosocial, biological, and behavioral characteristics that increase risk of developing cardiovascular disease.' As described in chapter 3, tryptophan depletion results in the expected increase in blood pressure and HPA activity. Muldoon et al. [85–87] showed that low serotonin responsivity to fenfluramine is associated with physical inactivity, greater body mass index, higher levels of triglycerides and glucose, greater insulin resistance, and preclinical arteriosclerosis. Similar effects were observed after challenge with citalopram, a highly selective SSRI.

Sleep disturbances: Sleep problems are prominent symptoms associated with stress, anxiety and depression. Antidepressants that block 5-HT_2 receptors have relatively strong effects on sleep maintenance [88]. The role of serotonin hypoactivity may only become relevant under chronic stress: recent data from Brummett et al. [89] suggest that sleep disturbances in carriers of the s-allele of the 5-HTTLPR are only present under stressful conditions.

Clearly, serotonin hypoactivity and hyporeactivity are associated with characteristic disturbances of mood, eating behavior, cognitive performance, sleep, metabolism, and cardiovascular function. Patterns of discrete psychological, biological, and symptom measures can be conceptualized to define such neuroendophenotypes. Although different serotonergic mechanisms account for these disturbances, a serotonin deficit seems to reflect a deficit of trophotropic function under stressful conditions, e.g. an inability to sufficiently protect the brain and the organism against ongoing demands.

7.2.4. Parasympathetic Hypoactivity and Hyporeactivity

Low parasympathetic activity has been reported to be relevant in some stress-related disorders. Basal vagal activity may be affected by genetic and epigenetic effects. Field et al. [27, 28] provided evidence on prenatal programming of low vagal tone in offspring of mothers who scored high on measures of anxiety, depression, and anger in the second trimester of pregnancy. Interestingly, these mothers also had a low vagal tone, possibly suggesting an ergotropic dominance in these subjects, which is genetically or epigenetically determined.

Parasympathetic hypoactivity has been proposed to be associated with functional bowel diseases [90]. In functional dyspepsia patients, low vagal tone seems to reduce antral motility under mental stress when compared to healthy test subjects [91]. Patients with atopic dermatitis had higher heart rate and lower vagal activity throughout the resting and stress phases under examination stress. They also scored significantly higher on measures of anxiety, depression and emotional excitability [92], suggesting an association of low vagal tone with mood.

Tougas [90] assumed that low vagal tone and increased sympathetic activity alter visceral perception. In patients with PTSD, a low vagal tone may account for deficient arousal and emotion regulation capacities often observed in PTSD. Sack et al. [93] observed decreased respiratory sinus arrhythmia (RSA) in response to a traumatic reminder and an association between low baseline RSA and sustained conditioned arousal in PTSD. In another experimental study in mice, Morgan et al. [94, p. 120] explored effects of vagal tone in healthy military personnel, exposed to a high-intensity military training. The authors observed a significant relationship between low vagal tone and superior performance, suggesting 'that vagal suppression is associated with enhanced performance under conditions of high stress and that this enhanced performance may be related to emotion regulation and cognitive functioning.' These data suggest an altered visceral perception in subjects or patients with low vagal tone, associated with characteristic emotional and cognitive changes.

Presently, the evidence of effects of parasympathetic hypoactivity and hyporeactivity on stress symptomatology is still anecdotal. However, it seems that an imbalance of sympathetic and parasympathetic activity can affect both visceral perception and disease vulnerability.

7.3. Summary

The serotonergic system plays a dominant role in the regulation of the stress response and stress-related disorders. Apart from multiple key functions of serotonin in brain development and bodily function, serotonergic fibers originating from the DR seem to exert important trophotropic functions in the adaptation to stress. These effects are clearly modified by environmental, genetic and epigenetic determinants. In this chapter, we tried to dissect the trophotropic serotonergic and parasympathetic effects, and to illustrate that a hypo- and hyperactivity or -reactivity of these systems results in characteristic endophenotypes, as described by alterations on psychological, biological, and symptom measures. However, unlike the noradrenergic system, trophotropic functions in the central nervous system are not dominated by a single system, but are far more complex and versatile. Their function to buffer ergotropic responses and to guarantee for recovery and reconstitution of brain physiology is obviously far more differentiated, allowing specific adaptation to actual needs and demands under stressful conditions. Today, we do not yet know the full spectrum of trophotropic mechanisms and functions.

References

1 Gellhorn E: The emotions and the ergotropic and trophotropic systems. Psychol Forsch 1970;34:48–94.

2 Ellison GD: Behavior and the balance between norepinephrine and serotonin. Acta Neurobiol Exp 1975;35:499–515.

3 Needham CW, Dila CJ: Synchronizing and desynchronizing systems of the old brain. Brain Res 1968; 11:285–293.

4 Kostowski W: Two noradrenergic systems in the brain and their interactions with other monoaminergic neurons. Polish J Pharmacol Pharmacy 1979; 31:425–436.

5 Massari VJ, Tizabi Y, Jacobowitz DM: Potential noradrenergic regulation of serotonergic neurons in the median raphe nucleus. Exp Brain Res 1979; 34:177–182.

6 McEwen BS: Physiology and neurobiology of stress and adaptation: central role of the brain. Physiol Rev 2007;87:873–904.

7 Charney DS: Psychobiological mechanisms of resilience and vulnerability: implications for successful adaptation to extreme stress. Am J Psychiatry 2004;161:195–216.

8 Hornung JP: The human raphe nuclei and the serotonergic system. J Chem Neuroanat 2003;26:331–343.

9 Kaehler ST, Singewald N, Philippu A: Dependence of serotonin release in the locus coeruleus on dorsal raphe neuronal activity. Naunyn-Schmiedeberg's Arch Pharmacol 1999;359:386–393.

10 Lopez JF, Vazquez DM, Chalmers DT, Watson SJ: Regulation of 5-HT receptors and the hypothalamic-pituitary-adrenal axis. Implications for the neurobiology of suicide. Ann NY Acad Sci 1997;836: 106–134.

11 Tanaka M, Yoshida M, Emoto H, Ishii H: Noradrenaline systems in the hypothalamus, amygdala and locus coeruleus are involved in the provocation of anxiety: basic studies. Eur J Pharmacol 2000;405: 397–406.

12 Chaouloff F, Berton O, Mormede P: Serotonin and stress. Neuropsychopharmacology 1999;21(2 suppl):28S–32S.

13 Caspi A, Sugden K, Moffitt TE, Taylor A, Craig IW, Harrington H, McClay J, Mill J, Martin J, Braithwaite A, Poulton R: Influence of life stress on depression: moderation by a polymorphism in the 5-HTT gene. Science 2003;301:386–389.

14 Serretti A, Benedetti F, Zanardi R, Smeraldi E: The influence of Serotonin Transporter Promoter Polymorphism (SERTPR) and other polymorphisms of the serotonin pathway on the efficacy of antidepressant treatments. Prog Neuro-Psychopharmacol Biol Psychiatry 2005;29:1074–1084.

15 Ebstein RP: The molecular genetic architecture of human personality: beyond self-report questionnaires. Mol Psychiatry 2006;11:427–445.

16 Smits KM, Smits LJ, Schouten JS, Stelma FF, Nelemans P, Prins MH: Influence of SERTPR and STin2 in the serotonin transporter gene on the effect of selective serotonin reuptake inhibitors in depression: a systematic review. Mol Psychiatry 2004;9: 433–441.

17 Wilhelm K, Siegel JE, Finch AW, Hadzi-Pavlovic D, Mitchell PB, Parker G, Schofield PR: The long and the short of it: associations between 5-HTT genotypes and coping with stress. Psychosom Med 2007; 69:614–620.

18 Wurtman RJ: Genes, stress, and depression. Metabolism 2005;54(5 suppl 1):16–19.

19 Hariri AR, Drabant EM, Munoz KE, Kolachana BS, Mattay VS, Egan MF, Weinberger DR: A susceptibility gene for affective disorders and the response of the human amygdala. Archs Gen Psychiatry 2005;62:146–152.

20 Levinson DF: The genetics of depression: a review. Biol Psychiatry 2006;60:84–92.

21 Nakhost A, Houeland G, Castellucci VF, Sossin WS: Differential regulation of transmitter release by alternatively spliced forms of synaptotagmin I. J Neurosci 2003;23:6238–6244.

22 Smith GS, Lotrich FE, Malhotra AK, Lee AT, Ma Y, Kramer E, Gregersen PK, Eidelberg D, Pollock BG: Effects of serotonin transporter promoter polymorphisms on serotonin function. Neuropsychopharmacology 2004;29:2226–2234.

23 Svenningsson P, Chergui K, Rachleff I, Flajolet M, Zhang X, El Yacoubi M, Vaugeois JM, Nomikos GG, Greengard P: Alterations in 5-HT1B receptor function by p11 in depression-like states. Science 2006; 311:77–80.

24 Moses-Kolko EL, Bogen D, Perel J, Bregar A, Uhl K, Levin B, Wisner KL: Neonatal signs after late in utero exposure to serotonin reuptake inhibitors: literature review and implications for clinical applications. JAMA 2005;293:2372–2383.

25 Whitaker-Azmitia PM: Behavioral and cellular consequences of increasing serotonergic activity during brain development: a role in autism? Int J Dev Neurosci 2005;23:75–83.

26 Gardner KL, Thrivikraman KV, Lightman SL, Plotsky PM, Lowry CA: Early life experience alters behavior during social defeat: focus on serotonergic systems. Neuroscience 2005;136:181–191.

27 Field T, Diego M, Hernandez-Reif M, Salman F, Schanberg S, Kuhn C, Yando R, Bendell D: Prenatal anger effects on the fetus and neonate. J Obstet Gynaecol 2002;22:260–266.

28 Field T, Diego M, Hernandez-Reif M, Schanberg S, Kuhn C, Yando R, Bendell D: Pregnancy anxiety and comorbid depression and anger: effects on the fetus and neonate. Depress Anxiety 2003;17:140–151.

29 Mandelli L, Serretti A, Marino E, Pirovano A, Calati R, Colombo C: Interaction between serotonin transporter gene, catechol-O-methyltransferase gene and stressful life events in mood disorders. Int J Neuropsychopharmacol 2007;10:437–447.

30 Vergne DE, Nemeroff CB: The interaction of serotonin transporter gene polymorphisms and early adverse life events on vulnerability for major depression. Curr Psychiatry Rep 2006;8:452–457.

31 Bondy B: Common genetic factors for depression and cardiovascular disease. Dialogues Clin Neurosci 2007;9:19–28.

32 Craig IW: The importance of stress and genetic variation in human aggression. Bioessays 2007;29: 227–236.

33 Birmingham DJ, Nagaraja HN, Rovin BH, Spetie L, Zhao Y, Li X, Hackshaw KV, Yu CY, Malarkey WB, Hebert LA: Fluctuation in self-perceived stress and increased risk of flare in patients with lupus nephritis carrying the serotonin receptor 1A -1019 G allele. Arthritis Rheum 2006;54:3291–3299.

34 Lee HJ, Lee MS, Kang RH, Kim H, Kim SD, Kee BS, Kim YH, Kim YK, Kim JB, Yeon BK, Oh KS, Oh BH, Yoon JS, Lee C, Jung HY, Chee IS, Paik IH: Influence of the serotonin transporter promoter gene polymorphism on susceptibility to posttraumatic stress disorder. Depress Anxiety 2005;21:135–139.

35 Maier SF, Watkins LR: Stressor controllability and learned helplessness: the roles of the dorsal raphe nucleus, serotonin, and corticotropin-releasing factor. Neurosci Biobehav Rev 2005;29:829–841.

36 Bethea CL, Lu NZ, Gundlah C, Streicher JM: Diverse actions of ovarian steroids in the serotonin neural system. Front Neuroendocrinol 2002;23:41–100.

37 Shively CA, Bethea CL: Cognition, mood disorders, and sex hormones. ILAR J 2004;45:189–199.

38 Raul L: Serotonin2 receptors in the nucleus tractus solitarius: characterization and role in the baroreceptor reflex arc. Cell Mol Neurobiol 2003;23:709–726.

39 Bauer M, Heinz A, Whybrow PC: Thyroid hormones, serotonin and mood: of synergy and significance in the adult brain. Mol Psychiatry 2002;7: 140–156.

40 Reif A, Lesch KP: Toward a molecular architecture of personality. Behav Brain Res 2003;139:1–20.

41 Hansson SR, Mezey E, Hoffman BJ: Serotonin transporter messenger RNA in the developing rat brain: early expression in serotonergic neurons and transient expression in non-serotonergic neurons. Neuroscience 1998;83:1185–1201.

42 Williams RB, Marchuk DA, Gadde KM, Barefoot JC, Grichnik K, Helms MJ, Kuhn CM, Lewis JG, Schanberg SM, Stafford-Smith M, Suarez EC, Clary GL, Svenson IK, Siegler IC: Central nervous system serotonin function and cardiovascular responses to stress. Psychosom Med 2001;63:300–305.

43 Overmier JB, Hellhammer DH: The learned helplessness model of human depression; in Simon P, Soubrie P, Widlocher D (eds): Animal Models in Psychiatric Disorders. Basel, Karger, 1988, pp 177–202.

44 Overmier JB, Leaf RC: Effects of discriminative Pavlovian fear conditioning upon previously or subsequently acquired avoidance responding. J Comp Physiol Psychol 1965;60:213–217.

45 Seligman MEP: Helplessness: On Depression, Development, and Death, ed 2. New York, Freeman, 1991.

46 Engel GL, Schmale AH: Conservation-withdrawal: a primary regulatory process for organismic homeostasis. Ciba Found Symp 1972;8:57–75.

47 Hellhammer DH: Learned helplessness – an animal model revisited; in Angst J (ed): The Origins of Depression: Current Concepts and Approaches. Berlin, Springer, 1983, pp 405–423.

48 Kalin NH, Shelton SE, Fox AS, Oakes TR, Davidson RJ: Brain regions associated with the expression and contextual regulation of anxiety in primates. Biol Psychiatry 2005;58:796–804.

49 Adell A, Garcia-Marquez C, Armario A, Gelpi E: Chronic stress increases serotonin and noradrenaline in rat brain and sensitizes their responses to a further acute stress. J Neurochem 1988;50:1678–1681.

50 Jezova D, Duncko R: Enhancement of stress-induced pituitary hormone release and cardiovascular activation by antidepressant treatment in healthy men. J Psychopharmacol (Oxford, England) 2002;16:235–240.

51 Hellhammer DH, Rea MA, Bell M, Belkien L, Ludwig M: Learned helplessness. Effects on brain monoamines and the pituitary-gonadal axis. Pharmacol Biochem Behav 1984;21:481–485.

52 Hellhammer DH: Gehirn und Verhalten. Eine anwendungsorientierte Einführung in die Psychobiologie. Münster, Aschendorff, 1983.

53 Peroutka SJ: 5-Hydroxytryptamine receptor subtypes: molecular, biochemical and physiological characterization. Trends Neurosci 1988;11:496–500.

54 Richardson BP, Engel G: The pharmacology and function of 5-HT3 receptors. Trends Neurosci 1986;9:424–428.

55 Vaddadi G, Lambert E, Corcoran SJ, Esler MD: Postural syncope: mechanisms and management. MJA 2007;187:299–304.

56 Hamer M, Steptoe A: Association between physical fitness, parasympathetic control, and proinflammatory responses to mental stress. Psychosom Med 2007;69:660–666.
57 Dorr AE, Debonnel G: Effect of vagus nerve stimulation on serotonergic and noradrenergic transmission. J Pharmacol Exp Ther 2006;318:890–898.
58 Nemeroff CB, Mayberg HS, Krahl SE, McNamara J, Frazer A, Henry TR, George MS, Charney DS, Brannan SK: VNS therapy in treatment-resistant depression: clinical evidence and putative neurobiological mechanisms. Neuropsychopharmacology 2006;31:1345–1355.
59 Hirschfeld RM, Montgomery SA, Keller MB, Kasper S, Schatzberg AF, Moller HJ, Healy D, Baldwin D, Humble M, Versiani M, Montenegro R, Bourgeois M: Social functioning in depression: a review. J Clin Psychiatry 2000;61:268–275.
60 Maes M, Meltzer YH: The Serotonin Hypothesis of Major Depression; in Bloom EF, Kupfer JD (eds): Psychopharmacology: The Fourth Generation of Progress. New York, Raven Press, 1995, pp 933–944.
61 Nemeroff CB: Recent advances in the neurobiology of depression. Psychopharmacol Bull 2002; 36(suppl 2):6–23.
62 Charmandari E, Kino T, Souvatzoglou E, Chrousos GP: Pediatric stress: hormonal mediators and human development. Horm Res 2003;59:161–179.
63 Heim C, Plotsky PM, Nemeroff CB: Importance of studying the contributions of early adverse experience to neurobiological findings in depression. Neuropsychopharmacology 2004;29:641–648.
64 Pace TW, Mletzko TC, Alagbe O, Musselman DL, Nemeroff CB, Miller AH, Heim CM: Increased stress induced inflammatory responses in male patients with major depression and increased early life stress. Am J Psychiatry 2006;163:1630–1633.
65 Kent JM, Coplan JD, Gorman JM: Clinical utility of the selective serotonin reuptake inhibitors in the spectrum of anxiety. Biol Psychiatry 1998;44:812–824.
66 Neumeister A, Bain E, Nugent AC, Carson RE, Bonne O, Luckenbaugh DA, Eckelman W, Herscovitch P, Charney DS, Drevets WC: Reduced serotonin type 1A receptor binding in panic disorder. J Neurosci 2004;24:589–591.
67 Gross C, Zhuang X, Stark K, Ramboz S, Oosting R, Kirby L, Santarelli L, Beck S, Hen R: Serotonin1A receptor acts during development to establish normal anxiety-like behaviour in the adult. Nature 2002;416:396–400.
68 Nutt DJ: Overview of diagnosis and drug treatments of anxiety disorders. CNS Spectrums 2005; 10:49–56.
69 Xu K, Ernst M, Goldman D: Imaging genomics applied to anxiety, stress response, and resiliency. Neuroinformatics 2006;4:51–64.
70 Kaplan A, Hollander E: A review of pharmacologic treatments for obsessive-compulsive disorder. Psychiatr Services (Washington, DC) 2003;54:1111–1118.
71 Delgado PL, Moreno FA: Different roles for serotonin in anti-obsessional drug action and the pathophysiology of obsessive-compulsive disorder. Br J Psychiatry 1998;35:21–25.
72 Talbot PS: The molecular neuroimaging of anxiety disorders. Curr Psychiatry Rep 2004;6:274–279.
73 Haller J, Mikics E, Halasz J, Toth M: Mechanisms differentiating normal from abnormal aggression: glucocorticoids and serotonin. Eur J Pharmacol 2005;526:89–100.
74 Summers CH, Winberg S: Interactions between the neural regulation of stress and aggression. J Exp Biol 2006;209:4581–4589.
75 Chamberlain SR, Sahakian BJ: The neuropsychiatry of impulsivity. Curr Opin Psychiatry 2007;20: 255–261.
76 Bell CJ, Hood SD, Nutt DJ: Acute tryptophan depletion. II. Clinical effects and implications. Aust NZ J Psychiatry 2005;39:565–574.
77 Talbot PS, Watson DR, Barrett SL, Cooper SJ: Rapid tryptophan depletion improves decision-making cognition in healthy humans without affecting reversal learning or set shifting. Neuropsychopharmacology 2006;31:1519–1525.
78 Chamberlain SR, Muller U, Robbins TW, Sahakian BJ: Neuropharmacological modulation of cognition. Curr Opin Neurol 2006;19:607–612.
79 Heninger GR, Delgado PL, Charney DS, Price LH, Aghajanian GK: Tryptophan-deficient diet and amino acid drink deplete plasma tryptophan and induce a relapse of depression in susceptible patients. J Chem Neuroanat 1992;5:347–348.
80 Landen M, Thase ME: A model to explain the therapeutic effects of serotonin reuptake inhibitors: the role of 5-HT2 receptors. Psychopharmacol Bull 2006;39:147–166.
81 Steiner M, Pearlstein T, Cohen LS, Endicott J, Kornstein SG, Roberts C, Roberts DL, Yonkers K: Expert guidelines for the treatment of severe PMS, PMDD, and comorbidities: the role of SSRIs. J Women's Health 2006;15:57–69.
82 Halford JC, Harrold JA, Boyland EJ, Lawton CL, Blundell JE: Serotonergic drugs: effects on appetite expression and use for the treatment of obesity. Drugs 2007;67:27–55.
83 Takeda E, Terao J, Nakaya Y, Miyamoto K, Baba Y, Chuman H, Kaji R, Ohmori T, Rokutan K: Stress control and human nutrition. J Med Invest 2004;51: 139–145.

84 Williams RB: Lower central nervous system serotonergic function and risk of cardiovascular disease: where are we, what's next? Stroke 2007;38:2213–2214.
85 Muldoon MF, Mackey RH, Korytkowski MT, Flory JD, Pollock BG, Manuck SB: The metabolic syndrome is associated with reduced central serotonergic responsivity in healthy community volunteers. J Clin Endocrinol Metab 2006;91:718–721.
86 Muldoon MF, Mackey RH, Sutton-Tyrrell K, Flory JD, Pollock BG, Manuck SB: Lower central serotonergic responsivity is associated with preclinical carotid artery atherosclerosis. Stroke 2007;38:2228–2233.
87 Muldoon MF, Mackey RH, Williams KV, Korytkowski MT, Flory JD, Manuck SB: Low central nervous system serotonergic responsivity is associated with the metabolic syndrome and physical inactivity. J Clin Endocrinol Metab 2004;89:266–271.
88 Thase ME: Depression and sleep: pathophysiology and treatment. Dialogues Clin Neurosci 2006;8:217–226.
89 Brummett BH, Krystal AD, Ashley-Koch A, Kuhn CM, Zuchner S, Siegler IC, Barefoot JC, Ballard EL, Gwyther LP, Williams RB: Sleep quality varies as a function of 5-HTTLPR genotype and stress. Psychosom Med 2007;69:621–624.
90 Tougas G: The autonomic nervous system in functional bowel disorders. Can J Gastroenterol 1999; 13(suppl A):15A–17A.
91 Hausken T, Svebak S, Wilhelmsen I, Haug TT, Olafsen K, Pettersson E, Hveem K, Berstad A: Low vagal tone and antral dysmotility in patients with functional dyspepsia. Psychosom Med 1993;55:12–22.
92 Seiffert K, Hilbert E, Schaechinger H, Zouboulis CC, Deter HC: Psychophysiological reactivity under mental stress in atopic dermatitis. Dermatology 2005;210:286–293.
93 Sack M, Hopper JW, Lamprecht F: Low respiratory sinus arrhythmia and prolonged psychophysiological arousal in posttraumatic stress disorder: heart rate dynamics and individual differences in arousal regulation. Biol Psychiatry 2004;55:284–290.
94 Morgan CA 3rd, Aikins DE, Steffian G, Coric V, Southwick S: Relation between cardiac vagal tone and performance in male military personnel exposed to high stress: three prospective studies. Psychophysiology 2007;44:120–127.

Subject Index